MANAGED CARE IN DENTISTRY

MANAGED CARE IN DENTISTRY

by
Bryan Quattlebaum, D.D.S.

PennWell Books

DENTAL ECONOMICS

PennWell Publishing Company
Tulsa, Oklahoma

Copyright © 1995 by
PennWell Publishing Company
1421 South Sheridan/P.O. Box 1260
Tulsa, Oklahoma 74101

Quattlebaum, Bryan.
    Managed care in dentistry/Bryan Quattlebaum.
    p.   cm.
    Includes bibliographical reference and index.
    ISBN 0-87814-433-1
    1. Managed dental health care—United States. I. Title.
    [DNLM: 1. Insurance, Dental—economics—United States. 2. Managed-Care Programs—organization & administration—United States. 3. Practice Management, Dental—organization & administration. 4. Dental Health Services—organization & administration—United States. W 275 AA1 Q18m 1994]
RK58.5.Q38   1994
362.1'976—dc20
DNLM/DLC
for Library of Congress   94-23729
                                                                                                                    CIP

All rights reserved. No part of this book may be reproduced, stored in a retrieval system, or transcribed in any form or by any means, electronic or mechanical, including photocopying and recording, without the prior written permission of the publisher.

Printed in the United States of America

1 2 3 4 5 99 98 97 96 95

DEDICATION

To my lovely and loving wife Lisa Renee—
you took a soul that was nearly empty
and poured the best of life back in. . .

CONTENTS

ACKNOWLEDGMENTS • viii

INTRODUCTION • ix

CHAPTER 1
You Have Nothing to Fear... and Everything to Understand • 1

CHAPTER 2
The Many Faces of Dental Plans • 14

CHAPTER 3
Surviving Health Care Reform: Today and Beyond • 26

CHAPTER 4
What Is Managed Care in Dentistry? • 36

CHAPTER 5
Quality Assurance and Dental Managed Care • 49

Contents

CHAPTER 6
Encounter Data Reporting—A Farewell to Claims • 58

CHAPTER 7
Provider Networks—IPAs and the Like • 67

CHAPTER 8
Special Concerns for the Dental Specialist • 87

CHAPTER 9
Making Room for Managed Care in Your Practice • 93

CHAPTER 10
Before You Join: 15 Questions You Must Ask of Every Plan • 100

CHAPTER 11
Provider Agreements—Making the Decision • 113

CHAPTER 12
Fractional Practice Analysis • 124

CHAPTER 13
*Dropouts—Dealing with Termination
from a Dental Managed-Care Program • 133*

CHAPTER 14
A Final Word • 138

APPENDIX I
The Knox-Keene Dental Guidelines • 141

APPENDIX II
A Sample Dental Provider Agreement • 173

GLOSSARY • 193

REFERENCES • 207

INDEX • 210

Acknowledgments

This book is a labor of many hours of research and reflection. Special thanks to the entire Dental Managed Care Unit (my "team") at the California Department of Health Services for simply being the best. All of the graphical content of this book is the work of my wife, Lisa, to whom this book is dedicated. My colleague and dear friend, Dr. Gertrude Paxton, devised the facility checklist and record review forms that added so much to this book.

To Richard Ryan of Dental Management Decisions, for the inspiration behind "Fractional Practice Analysis." Richard is who *I* go to for advice about managed care.

To my ever-patient editor at PennWell, Jaree McNamara, without whose patience and guidance the opportunity to publish this book would remain a dream.

And a special acknowledgment of a man who, during my residency in periodontics at the Naval Dental School, taught me how to think, write, and perform research in a way that changed my life forever—Dr. James Mellonig.

INTRODUCTION

"If economists could manage to get themselves thought of as humble, competent people on a level with dentists, that would be splendid."

JOHN MAYNARD KEYNES (1883–1946), BRITISH ECONOMIST. "THE FUTURE," *ESSAYS IN PERSUASION* (1931) FROM *THE COLUMBIA DICTIONARY OF QUOTATIONS* (COLUMBIA UNIVERSITY PRESS, 1993).

In reality, my friend, this book is a journey.

Never in my wildest dreams would I have envisioned myself, hands trembling while attempting my first dental school crown wax-up, that one day I would be authoring a book on a subject that has caused many of my own colleagues' hands to tremble again.

The subject is dental managed care. It is a very real part of our profession, and while our medical colleagues are about a decade ahead of us in experience, the clamor over national health-care reform during

Table I-1
Projected Managed Care Growth.

	1990	1995	2000
HMO	15%	25%	50%
POS/PPO	25%	40%	35%
Traditional	35%	15%	0%

[Source: Blue Cross Blue Shield of Illinios (New York: Dental Managed Care Congress, 1994)]

the Clinton administration is forcing all dentists to learn about dental managed care, and learn it now (see Table I–1).

When I took the Dental Admission Test in 1974, dentistry existed in a very different world. Dentists who advertised in the Yellow Pages were in a small minority that were branded "credit dentists" and were shunned from membership in most organized dental societies. Young graduates were often advised by their dental school mentors to set up practices in areas conducive to the good life—"the patients will find you." In reality, the local banks found you first and were ready and willing to fund the new dentist in town.

How different a world the dental profession finds itself in today. Dentists advertise on bus benches and on television—competition for patients is fierce. Federal agencies with acronyms such as FTC and OSHA have made profound changes on the profession of dentistry. They continue to do so.

As for myself, I (unwittingly) embarked upon a very dynamic career in dentistry. Upon graduation from the University of the Pacific School of Dentistry in 1979, I was in general practice in San Francisco for nearly a year until a spot opened up for me in the U.S. Navy Dental Corps. I had always planned to perform some military service as a dentist, for I felt my professional skills were embryonic, and the military offered a wealth of experience.

My career with the U.S. Navy was a very special one for me. I traveled the Pacific Rim nations aboard the USS *Kitty Hawk (CV-63)*, an aging but highly capable aircraft carrier. The naval submarine base in Bangor, Washington, introduced me to the silent service—those submariners of the (then) brand-new Trident missile boats. From there, I was selected for specialty training in periodontics at Bethesda, Maryland, under the superb tutelage of Dr. James Mellonig.

Introduction

My "payback period" for the periodontics residency ended in San Diego in 1989. After a year in private practice and teaching, I became a senior consultant for Government Programs with Delta Dental Plan of California. This position was held for nearly three years before I progressed to my present position as chief dental consultant, Dental Managed Care Unit of the California Department of Health Services.

Looking back upon my career, I marvel at both the diversity and good fortune that awaited me. Dental school taught me dentistry. Private practice taught me the integration of business principles with running a professional office (all too often the hard way). The U.S. Navy taught me the administrative skills needed for large-scale clinical practice, along with much of what was really dental managed care. Government service was also my first introduction to the various internal quality assurance programs (e.g., Total Quality Management, Continuous Quality Improvement, etc.), along with credentialing, privileging, and coordinated case management of patients with colleagues in medicine and allied heath programs.

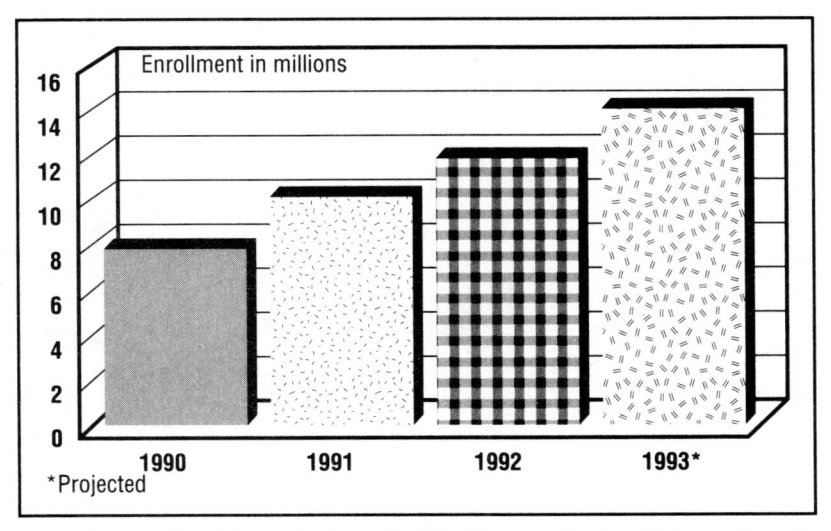

Figure I–1. Enrollment in dental HMOs [Source: National Association of Prepaid Dental Plans, 1992 Survey (Dallas: National Association of Prepaid Dental Plans, 1993)]

My time at Delta Dental Plan of California taught me the very different world of dental service plan administration. My involvement included the extremely volatile Denti-Cal program, once an entirely fee-for-service-based Medicaid program that will soon give way to the largest dental managed-care program of its kind—the Medi-Cal Dental Managed Care Program. It is with and by these diverse credentials that I find myself immersed in dental managed care.

Dental managed care must not be ignored. The National Association of Prepaid Dental Plans (NAPDP) reported that enrollment in dental managed-care plans reached 10.4 million in 1991, an increase of 25% from the previous year[1] (see Fig. I–1). By the time you read the first edition of this book, enrollment may top 15 million. Prestigious firms such as Hewlett-Packard have found dramatic savings and ample employee satisfaction in dental managed care, and not a single workday goes by without another dental managed-care program having been sold to corporate America.

Dental managed care is here to stay. We can choose to ignore it or we can work to understand it. By continuing this journey with me, I will know that you have wisely chosen the latter.

CHAPTER 1

YOU HAVE NOTHING TO FEAR... AND EVERYTHING TO UNDERSTAND

"The man who has ceased to fear has ceased to care."
F.H. BRADLEY (1846–1924), ENGLISH PHILOSOPHER. *APHORISMS*, NO. 63 (1930) FROM *THE COLUMBIA DICTIONARY OF QUOTATIONS* (COLUMBIA UNIVERSITY PRESS, 1993).

"If one does not understand a person, one tends to regard him as a fool."
CARL JUNG (1875–1961), SWISS PSYCHIATRIST. "MYSTERIUM CONIUNCTIONIS," ED. WILLIAM MCGUIRE, VOL. 14, REPRINTED IN *COLLECTED WORKS* (1963) FROM *THE COLUMBIA DICTIONARY OF QUOTATIONS* (COLUMBIA UNIVERSITY PRESS, 1993).

It is in our very nature, not just as dental professionals but also as human beings, to initially fear that which is unknown to us. It is not the fault of any individual dentist, nor dental institution, that we have relegated ourselves largely to solo practice—not availing ourselves of the "other" dental practice environments that many believe we will be forced into by the spectre of dental managed care. The various alternatives to solo private practice have proven satisfactory to many American dentists and are not inherently inferior. Some of you, after reading this book, may find these alternative choices more attractive than you ever thought was possible.

In the preface to *The President's Health Security Plan,* Erik Eckholm of the *New York Times* captures this sentiment wonderfully. As he tells it:

> *In a field rife with special interests, nearly every organized group has complained, even those that stand to gain from the proposals. Large corporations welcome the prospect of strong cost controls, but bemoan the new regulations to which they would have to adhere. The larger insurance companies, which have already begun developing managed care plans, would presumably thrive under the system but they attack the proposed budget caps as pernicious. Doctors support extending generous insurance to everyone, which means 37 million new paying patients. But they lament the pressures that will push most of them and their new patients into managed care plans, which limit their autonomy, they resent proposed restrictions on fees and they fear the impact of overall budget limits.*[2]

The queasiness about managed care in dentistry is not the exclusive domain of the dentist. When the Los Angeles Unified School District changed from a fee-for-service plan to a managed-care (capitation) plan on January 1, 1993, a study by the California Dental Association found that "91% of employees were satisfied with the fee-for-service plan but only 17% of those aware of the change were satisfied with the new prepaid plan" (see Fig. 1–1).[3]

It is interesting to note that the study implies that a sizable

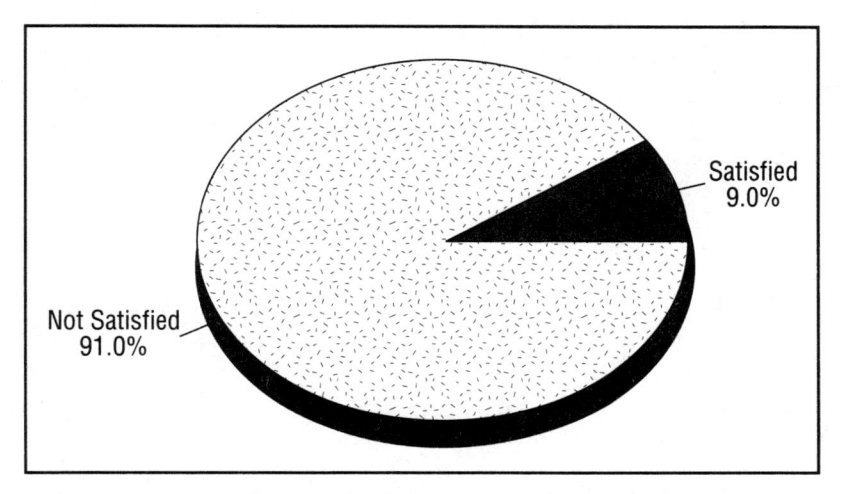

Figure 1-1. L.A.U.S.D. employee satisfaction (FFS to HMO) [Source: California Dental Association (Sacramento: California Dental Association, 1993)]

percentage of the employees were not even aware that they had lost their fee-for-service option. A follow-up study being conducted by the California Dental Association is finding a significant increase in patient satisfaction has taken place over time.

Why are the changes happening in the first place? Our nation is faced with one out of every seven citizens going without health insurance of any kind over an entire year. The numbers grow by 100,000 per month, and 128 million citizens are specifically without dental coverage of any kind.

Moreover, 63% of health-care coverage for Americans is job-based, employer-purchased benefit packages. These purchasers are demanding value for their purchasing dollars, and both employer and employee fear that the price tag for health care is increasing in an uncontrollable fashion.

Fear of rising health-care costs is ubiquitous. People are discussing the situation in many places, including the "cyberspace." Most of the on-line computer services today have areas of open discussions or forums. Any service member can make a comment or express an idea. Another member, perhaps at another time, can answer—to avoid everyone's contributions becoming gibberish, the master system forms a "thread." I found such a thread one night, and entered the commands that allowed me to follow the conversations from their initial comments to an eventual close. Because it deals with the issue of costs, I offer an edited version of it below (names have been changed):

To: All

From: Barbara

I'd like to know WHY a dentist has to look in my mouth after every cleaning? Is it required by law? And then have the dentist charge an extra $35 for it?

To: Barbara

From: Dr. Jim

A cleaning or prophylaxis without an exam is a service done out of context. I would be wary of any dentist that did not want to examine your teeth after a cleaning was performed.

To: Dr. Jim

From: Barbara

Thank you for your answer. I can understand what you said about having an exam. I do, however, think the cost should be included. I think in my next life, however, I should have a dentist in the family!

To: Barbara

From: Dr. Jim

I feel that I have to try and correct your perceptions about the cost of dental care. The overhead of a dental practice is high! Around 65%. It costs somewhere between $15–$20 just to have a treatment room ready for a new patient.

    I have two children who are always going to the pediatrician for something. If they are examined briefly and given an Rx, I pay about $60. No one bats an eye at this. But so many patients don't want to pay for dental care unless something is "done"!

To: Dr. Jim

From: Judy

Medical costs are a mystery to me. Personally, $60 for a brief doctor visit **would** make me bat an eye. The prices my current dentist charges seem reasonable enough, and I trust him, but it's really almost impossible to comparison shop. **I'm all for prices that provide a reasonable profit, but I have no understanding of why medical and dental fees are what they are.**

To: Dr. Jim

From: Dr. Stein

In my practice, my overheads are currently running at around 75%, with staff wages at 30%, equipment leasing/financing at 25%, and variables eating up the remainder. Currently, I work 36 hours chairside and at least 15–20 hours administration, and I feel that I am getting paid what I am worth (net). **However, one must never lose sight of the fact that since our patients pay our salaries, we are only able to be worth what the market will stand.**

Many dental professionals facing the current market realities of supply-and-demand have found that even the predominant "fee-for-service" dental programs did little to simplify dental office management. Regular filing of fees, enforcement of "favored nations" contractual clauses in participating provider agreements, increasing volumes and complexity of claim forms, delays in treatment authorizations—none of these elements of fee-for-service dentistry was ever considered "dentist-friendly."

In reality, every traditional "indemnity" product sold as a dental plan that had some element of fee-for-service (usual, customary, and reasonable fees on file, or prenegotiated reduced-fee schedules) in it still imposed cost containment methodologies in terms of:

- Benefit limitations and exclusions
- Annual deductibles
- Required patient co-payments determined by category of procedure

- Annual benefit ceilings (e.g., $1,000 in total dental fees paid per year)

These dental service program elements yield an Achilles' heel, for each model assumes that the dentist is setting fees based on a market-sensitive methodology. A methodology that, to a benefits manager, government agency, or small business owner, is analogous to price-setting methodologies commonly used in business and industry.

This is the fundamental reason why dental service plans are seeing their traditional products dry up and managed-care environments springing to life. There comes a point when, despite the fact that the dental profession has held its fees to a slower growth than the medical profession, the prudent purchaser asks the same question as our computer conversant—why are fees seemingly high? What determines that a crown should cost $500? *The purchaser of dental benefits is now demanding cost controls and (indirectly) pricing methodologies that have never before been imposed upon health professionals.*

The buyer of health-care benefits wants accountability in cost, as well as assurances that maximum *value* is being purchased for each dollar spent. In this quest, many providers of dental care perceive that a trade-off must be made between the quality of dental care delivered and cost containment. In reality, dental managed care proposes no such trade-off, for the following reasons:

- No inherent conflict must exist between quality standards and financial responsibility

- Improved quality of care is more easily obtainable when cost containment approaches reduce administrative burdens on available resources

- Cost-ineffective care is inherently of poor quality

Managed care is especially well-suited for purchasers seeking an appropriate balance between these two goals.

Dr. Molly Joel Coye, former director of the California Department of Health Services, is a world-renowned expert in health-care delivery systems. On this issue of accountability, she states, "Unlike fee-for-service, providers operating in a managed-care environment are formally and systematically linked in a manner that allows quality of care to be

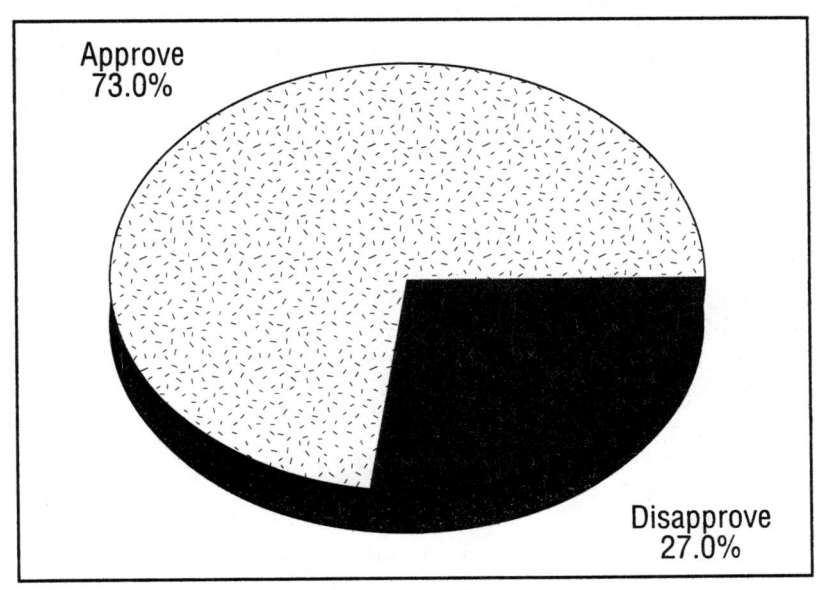

Figure 1-2. Parameters of care (response of AGD membership) (However, 77% of AGD members feared parameters would be used against them.) [Source: F.S. Foti, "Parameters of Care," *AGD Impact* 22, no. 3 (1994)]

rationally assessed and *accountability for care to be established and monitored*"4 (emphasis added).

Essential to the proper accounting and assessing of dental services is the existence of parameters of care. The American Dental Association defines dental parameters of care as "the range of appropriate treatment that can achieve a desired outcome. It represents alternatives for patient care and can be used to assist dentists in clinical decision-making. Parameters identify characteristics and components of quality patient care. They are neither minimal nor aspirational, but represent quality care commensurate with current scientific technology, knowledge, and resources. They provide guidance for a pattern of practice rather than for the care of a particular patient."5

The April 1994 issue of *AGD Impact,* the publication for the

Academy of General Dentistry, reported the following reaction of their membership to parameters of care (see Fig. 1–2):

> 73% of respondents indicated the dental profession should be involved in developing parameters of care for all conditions. AGD members who support involvement in the development of parameters of care for the profession most often believe that such parameters would encourage:

- continuing dental education
- decrease risk in delivering patient care
- help in therapeutic decisions
- hold all practitioners to one standard of care
- increase comfort in delivering of patient care

> More interesting was the observation that 77% of the AGD members supporting parameters of care also think that government agencies and third-party payment mechanisms will use them against the profession.[6]

For many years, organized dentistry feared the issuance of parameters. Even the California Dental Association, an early leader in helping to define quality dentistry with the publication of the pioneering *Quality Evaluation for Dental Care: Guidelines for the Assessment of Clinical Quality and Professional Performance,* stopped short of writing official parameters. And yet, the American Dental Association's own legal department reported in 1991 that "properly formulated parameters would not lead to increased malpractice exposure. In fact, properly formulated parameters should protect dentists who are practicing within a wide range of acceptable care."[7]

The American Dental Association still did not mount a serious effort until late spring of 1994. At that time, it was expected to reach completion in time for the 1994 House of Delegates session, set for October of that same year.

Dr. Albert Guay, a former member and chairman of the American Dental Association Council on Dental Care Programs, had this to say: "The development of parameters of care by the profession will be of great assistance in discouraging poorly designed or very restrictive plans. Plans will have to be designed that allow for the provision of adequate care. In fact, plan operators may well be subject to tort liability if they do not provide benefits for promised necessary care. Well-developed parameters of care can be used to define adequate care."[8]

Delta Dental Plan of Minnesota decided not to wait for organized dentistry to issue formal parameters of care. When the Minnesota legislature created that state's Integrated Service Networks, and Delta Dental Plan of Minnesota decided to enter the managed-care market, Dr. Tom Ireland, Delta's dental director, took the initiative. Standardized protocols were determined to be a key factor in Delta's strategy of developing quality managed-care programs in compliance with the new state laws. A panel of dentists ranging from practicing dentists to University of Minnesota's dental school professors was responsible for drafting the parameters. As Dr. Ireland stated, "If we are going to provide managed care, we have to have a baseline against which to decide what is appropriate. That's what the parameters will provide for us. Also, we want to make sure patients are getting appropriate care that is also cost-effective. That, in a nutshell, is the definition of value."[9]

Today's dentist must understand dental managed care. It is here to stay. While there may remain fiefdoms of fee-for-service dentistry scattered throughout the country, some form of managed care will exist. If we shy away from dental managed care, then we risk, as Dr. Jung admonished, being judged the fool.

Despite the start-up blues encountered by the L.A.U.S.D. discussed earlier, there is increasing evidence that dental managed care is working for groups and purchasers throughout the country.

The Chicago public schools faced a severe budget crisis in 1990. With more than 43,000 lives for which to provide benefits, Chicago opted for a dual-option plan, giving employees a choice between traditional dental coverage and a dental managed-care plan.

The dental managed-care (DMO) plan requires no deductible and covers 100% of services for the first $1,000 of dental care. After that, the DMO pays for all preventive and basic services, such as the restoration of cavities, 80% of cast crowns, and 50% of bridges and dentures. School employees pay no premiums for their own coverage, and within two years more than 24% opted for the DMO plan. The Chicago school system is saving money at the rate of $4 million/year.

The teachers' union of Florida's Dade County public school system has been a proponent of dental managed care since 1975. In fact, the school system's 30,000 employees are now choosing from two DMO plans and one indemnity plan. Employees pay nothing for their own coverage—family coverage is $15 per month for the DMO plan and $28 per month in the indemnity plan. Less than one-third of eligible employees sign up for the indemnity dental plan.

In other areas of the country, dental managed-care plans face difficult hurdles, mostly from dentists who fear managed care. One of the prime goals of this book is to allay that fear—for fear breeds inaction, and many providers have left the decision on whether to incorporate managed care into their practices until it was too late.

This is not to imply that dental managed-care plans seek retribution against dentists who initially refuse to join provider networks—it is merely a situation that once a managed-care network has contracted with sufficient numbers of providers for a given patient population, there simply isn't room for additional providers.

Managed care is also managed competition. In order to reduce costs, dental managed-care plans offer network providers:

- A larger patient base without direct marketing costs
- Valuable quality assessment input
- Steady monthly incomes

In return, equitable reimbursement agreements are negotiated (not fee-for-service). Managed care means developing provider networks that will provide accessibility to dental services and quality care **with the minimum number of providers necessary.**

Thus does the free market enter the world of dental practice. The free market can be a cold, hostile place, especially if you are a dentist shut out from managed care.

Don Shuwarger, M.D., is a medical colleague who was caught unawares when "managed care came to town." He related to me a situation that many providers fear, and there is much to learn from his story (reprinted here by permission):

Clear Lake is a bedroom community halfway between Houston and Galveston. The community is home to the Johnson Space Center of the National Aeronautics and Space Administration. It is a tranquil neighborhood with a low crime rate, high educational level, and access to varied recreational opportunities. It seemed, nine years ago, to be a perfect place to settle and set up practice.

My solo practice OB/GYN office grew quickly and I became involved in the community. As chair of the Clear Lake Chamber of Commerce task force on health care, we developed community outreach programs and health fairs. This community was everything for which I had hoped and was very accepting of me.

Managed care was something that, while always present in the community, was not a very significant factor in my practice. Most of the NASA subcontractors, nearby oil-related industries, and small businesses provided their employees with a choice of insurance programs. These ranged from traditional indemnity insurance to preferred provider organizations (PPO) to health maintenance organizations (HMO). While some larger group practices depended heavily on managed-care programs, my solo practice flourished without the need for participation in managed care. It's not that I didn't want to accept managed care, but rather there was no need to do so, and the office couldn't handle the additional patient volume and administrative load.

All that changed abruptly. In October 1993, it was announced that numerous NASA subcontractors were going to contract with only one particular insurer for HMO and PPO products. **The traditional indemnity policy was priced prohibitively, so few if any families could afford it.** *Many other medium-sized employers and oil industry firms followed their lead. Within a few weeks, there was going to be a drastic change in my patients' access to their health care.*

Patients called every day and asked us to participate in their plans.

It was apparent that if my patients' continuity of care and freedom of choice in health-care provider was to be preserved, I would need to participate with the major managed-care plans. Calls were made to the provider relations offices of Prudential, The Travelers, MetLife, and Aetna.

Our first surprise came when we received a terse letter from the Travelers. Thank you for your interest, it said, but they were unable to offer me an application. Then the same from Prudential. Yet another from MetLife. The final one from Aetna was crushing. Soon, more than 3,000 patients were to find themselves a new gynecologist because their managed-care plan was not willing to send me even an application.

Patients did not understand this. Many said they were told by the insurer and their company that they could ask their doctor to join or ask the company to contact their doctor to see if he was interested in joining their managed-care plan. Many patients told me that the insurer told them at company meetings that the managed-care plan only accepted physicians who were highly qualified. The impression left with my patients was that I must be less than qualified.

Confused, bewildered, hurt, and scared, I turned to the Texas Medical Association (TMA) for information. Their general counsel advised me that Texas state law requires PPO plans to provide physicians with a fair, reasonable, and equivalent opportunity to participate. He wrote letters to the four insurers for me, but received a verbal response from only one company. I wrote to the Texas Department of Insurance and received no reply.

Another flurry of calls to the TMA resulted in the suggestion that I contact as many of my patients as possible who had been affected by this situation. It was recommended that patients be asked to contact both their insurers and the Texas Department of Insurance and register their complaints. So far, there has been no action by the insurance department. Aetna did suggest that I could appeal their refusal to provide me an application. Such an appeal was filed, but it is laughable. How can I begin to provide an appeal of an arbitrary decision not based on anything within my control, such as training, experience, board certification, and the like? There has been no word from Aetna on my appeal.

The effects and implications of these insurance company exclusions have been profound for my patients, staff, and family. Literally thousands of patients have had to abruptly change physicians, often in the middle of treatment or pregnancy care. The volume of medical records copying and mailing is bogging down the staff and destroying morale. Patients are in tears about the disruption of their care and being forced to change physicians against their will. Certainly, they could continue to see me, but they have a $1,000 deductible and then only 60% coverage afterwards. When this is compared to no deductible and a $10 per visit co-payment, there is really no reasonably affordable option to see a physician out of their plan. My family and I are constantly being asked why I don't participate in these various plans. People are polite, but underneath their question is the unspoken doubt of my qualifications.

Physicians who are the victims of this type of arbitrary discrimination and exclusionary policies need to network together. Each separate physician can feel isolated, persecuted, and fearful. By sharing experiences with others who have been similarly affected, the sense of loneliness will abate. Also, by talking together we can learn if others have been successful in reversing this problem and what approaches they have used.[10]

CHAPTER 2

THE MANY FACES OF DENTAL PLANS

"Marriage is popular because it combines the maximum of temptation with the maximum of opportunity."

GEORGE BERNARD SHAW (1856–1950), ANGLO-IRISH PLAYWRIGHT, CRITIC. "MAXIMS FOR REVOLUTIONISTS: MARRIAGE," *MAN AND SUPERMAN* (1903) FROM *THE COLUMBIA DICTIONARY OF QUOTATIONS* (COLUMBIA UNIVERSITY PRESS, 1993).

OVERVIEW

Dental plans and managed care may seem to many as strange bedfellows. Reflecting upon the George Bernard Shaw quote, perhaps they represent a fitting marriage. In either case, this chapter presents an opportunity to analyze the various existing dental plan structures (see Fig. 2–1).

Dental plans do not truly represent "insurance." Much has been made of "indemnity" dental plans, but indemnity insurance policies are meant to cover losses suffered in a catastrophic event. Regularly recurring or common events, such as visiting the dentist for a recall examination, radiographs, and cleaning, would be an actuary's nightmare. Premiums would soar through the roof—assuming that the insurance company wanted to stay in business and realize a profit.

Although this book refers to "dental plans" as a generic term, a more complete description would be dental benefit program. These programs are typically designed so that:

- Groups, not individuals, are eligible to join
- Groups may have to show prior experience with a dental plan
- Individual providers do not share in underwriting risks (or plan profit)

These requirements safeguard against adverse selection—a situation in which the total population of insured fails to fall along a normal bell-shaped curve of low-to-medium-to-high utilizers of dental services. Individuals are not allowed to join, since the underlying assumption is that they would not be seeking coverage unless they felt that they needed it. The addition of these potentially high utilizers would skew the normal distribution of dental-care utilization towards which dental-plan administrators aim.

Fee-for-Service	Preferred Provider Organization	Dental Managed Care
UCR Fees	Fixed Fees	Prospective Payment
No Networks	Limited Panel	Provider Network
Claims Payment	Claims Payment	Encounter Data

Figure 2–1. Dental plan characteristics

A common complaint about managed-care plans is that they secretly "hope" that no one will utilize their services. Traditional dental benefit plans expect to have the services required by the high utilizers more than fully paid for by the lesser utilizers, since premium costs do not vary within the group. It is a fallacy to believe that both environments strive for **full** utilization of all available dental services without some sort of utilization review and control.

If a dental plan does suffer from adverse selection (a preponderance of high utilizers), then traditionally it has been the plan that bears the financial risk (loss). While managed-care plans in dentistry have various kinds of provider-reimbursement methods, the plans do place varying levels of financial risk directly on the provider. The most common of these is capitation, in which the provider (most commonly the primary care dentist) is assigned a group of patients and is reimbursed at a fixed dollar value per person per month. Medical plans often call this a "prospective" form of provider payment.

Organized dentistry has long fought the battle against capitation, preferring to free the dentist from any financial risk of underwriting and tying reimbursement to payment for services rendered, or fee-for-service (FFS). This type of payment is by nature retrospective, requiring the filing of claims for payment with the dental plan.

PAYMENT BASED ON UCR FEES

"UCR" refers to fees that are:

1. the charge the dentist would usually make to any patient for a given procedure,

2. the customary charge that dentists in the surrounding community would also make for the same procedure, and

3. a reasonable charge for the time, expertise, lab costs, etc., expended by the dentist during treatment.

In order to determine UCR fees, dentists must usually become participating providers with a plan and agree to file their fees periodically. As an industry standard, if any fee for a given procedure lies above the 80th percentile of a distribution of fees from other providers, that fee is deemed "excessive." Many dentists have been horrified to learn that patients have been notified directly by some dental plans of claim payment rejections because their dentist's fee was excessive.

From the patient's perspective, the dental benefit plan would typically call for an annual deductible of around $50 to be paid per person prior to the plan making any payments. Afterward, the plan might cover 80% to 100% of preventive and basic services, as well as about 50% of the cost of dentures, fixed prosthodontics, or other major dental work. Other benefits that could be vulnerable to high costs, such as temporomandibular joint (TMJ) therapy and dental implants, are generally excluded from coverage.

Finally, the typical dental plan will impose a maximum annual benefit of $500 to $1,000, making the indemnity fee-for-service plan closer to a payment assistance program for patients.

In promoting freedom of choice among participating providers, these dental plans have a diminished ability to manage costs, conduct quality assurance programs, and accomplish effective utilization management. There may be limited opportunity to have dental consultants perform a review of submitted claims. In all cases, professional reviews are retrospective in scope.

SCHEDULE OF MAXIMUM ALLOWANCES, TABLE OF ALLOWANCES, AND SCHEDULE OF BENEFITS

In these variants from UCR fees, the dental plan generally determines what fees it is willing to pay for each procedure. Participating dentists agree to charge plan members these prenegotiated fees as payment in full, or the plan may allow the dentist to engage in balance billing. Balance billing involves charging the patient any difference between what the plan agrees to pay and the dentist's UCR fees.

COST CONTAINMENT IN FEE-FOR-SERVICE PLANS

As a further means of limiting the financial risk of dental plans doing business in the FFS mode, the benefit plan may include the following additional charges paid by the patient:

- Annual deductibles
- Co-payments
- Annual benefit maximums (or "ceilings")

These plans universally require the dentist to collect these deductibles and co-payments from patients before billing the plan for services rendered. The fact that some dentists "forgive" these payments, or inform patients that whatever their dental plan pays will be accepted as "payment in full" is not a trifle act. Besides disrupting the cost containment strategy established by the dental plan, the end effect is usually inflationary—plans increase premiums to offset the higher costs in claims payments, and the dentists raise their fees to close the gap. This upward spiral is yet another justification to purchasers of health care to turn to managed-care plans for lower premiums and more effective forms of cost containment.

DIRECT REIMBURSEMENT

In the scenario of direct reimbursement, the semblance of fee-for-service is preserved without "having" to deal with a dental plan. The patient obtains dental services from a provider of his or her choice, the dentist collects directly from the patient, and the employer reimburses the patient. Many local and state dental organizations have heavily promoted direct reimbursement as a way of preserving fee-for-service, freedom-of-choice dentistry in the face of managed-care-oriented health-care reform.

The problem with direct reimbursement lies in the fact that this system provides the purchaser of services with virtually no accountability of the dental services rendered to the patient. There are no utilization controls or review process, no monitoring of provider abuse, no cost containment—in essence, the lack of those very elements that originally brought about the birth of dental benefit plans. Direct reimbursement is the poorest of all available alternatives to dental managed care, and offers nothing to help the purchaser determine quality of care and benefit value.

PREFERRED PROVIDER ORGANIZATIONS

PPOs are really a marketing tool for dental plans. They function by diverting FFS patients into selected offices that have negotiated reduced fees with the dental plan, often 20% to 25% less than a UCR-based system. The basic elements of a FFS dental plan remain—co-payments, deductibles, benefit maximums, filing of claim forms for payment—all the while imposing a limited panel of providers. In some variants, patients are allowed to see any dentist outside of the panel, but in doing so suffer much higher out-of-pocket expenses (see Fig. 2–2).

A vicious cycle can occur in PPO arrangements similar to direct reimbursement. The plan may need to resort to extensive audits and utilization management tactics to ensure that dentists are not overbilling to compensate for a lower fee schedule. The dentist may raise fees to patients of other plans in a "loss-leader" strategy, which eventually drives up all dental costs. The plans, faced with higher administrative costs, attempt to pass them on to the purchasers and patients themselves.

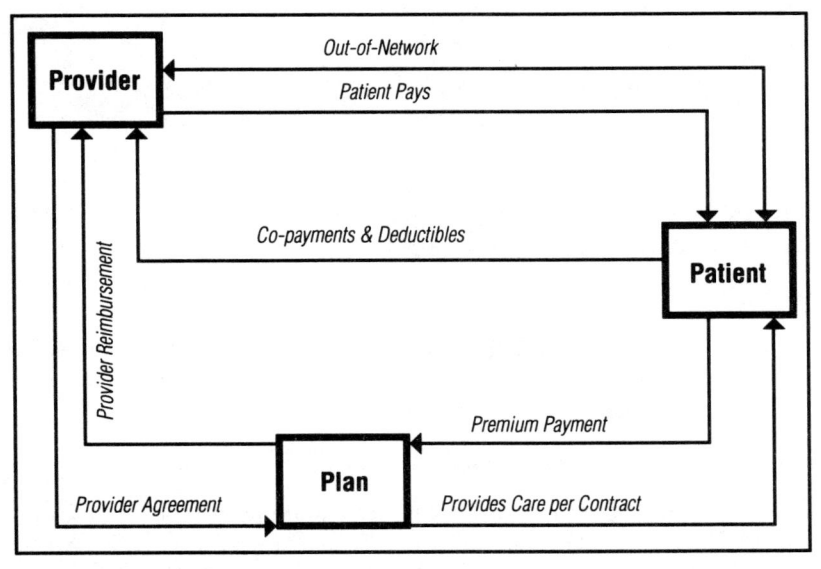

Figure 2–2. PPO systems

Another failing of PPOs is that very few actually pay claims. Any delay in claims processing and subsequent payments to providers cannot be readily dealt with by contacting the PPO. PPOs add an administrative layer that, while very effective at negotiations with dentists and the formation of provider networks, fails to achieve a level of accountability and control that today's free market is demanding.

EXCLUSIVE PROVIDER ORGANIZATIONS

Exclusive Provider Organizations? If the reader hasn't already guessed, these are exclusive panels of providers where no choice is given to patients outside the panel.

CAPITATION-BASED PROGRAMS

The first capitation-based dental plan was started in the early 1950s by Max Schoen, D.D.S. Dr. Schoen had been approached by the International Longshoremen's Union-Pacific Maritime Association in California. As Dr. Schoen reported:

> *When this author developed the capitation program of the ILWU-PMA children's dental plan for the Los Angeles area in 1953–1954, it included several principles as essential requirements for the achievement of the best possible oral-health status of the enrollees at a reasonable cost. Immediate goals:*
>
> - High utilization and completion of initial care
> - High utilization for regular maintenance care
>
> Methods to achieve goals:
>
> - Aggressive stimulation of regular use of care
> - Few exclusions, limitations, and co-payments
> - Capitation payment sufficient to cover average costs

- Care to be provided by broad-spectrum group practice with no intermediary
- Dentist participation in decision making
- Income based primarily on salary[11]

In a dental capitation program, per capita payments are made to network providers who assume full or partial risk for delivering a defined scope of benefits to a specified, assigned group of patients (see Fig. 2–3). In place of claim forms, "encounter data" is collected and analyzed by the dental plan, a function far less expensive than claims processing and review.

For the patient, less cost-shifting has to occur between low utilizers and high utilizers. For primary-care-level procedures, patients often face no out-of-pocket expenses. Only when higher cost, more extensive treatment is required might the patient incur expense—and then generally at a reduced fee schedule.

A totally capitated reimbursement program is virtually nonexistent

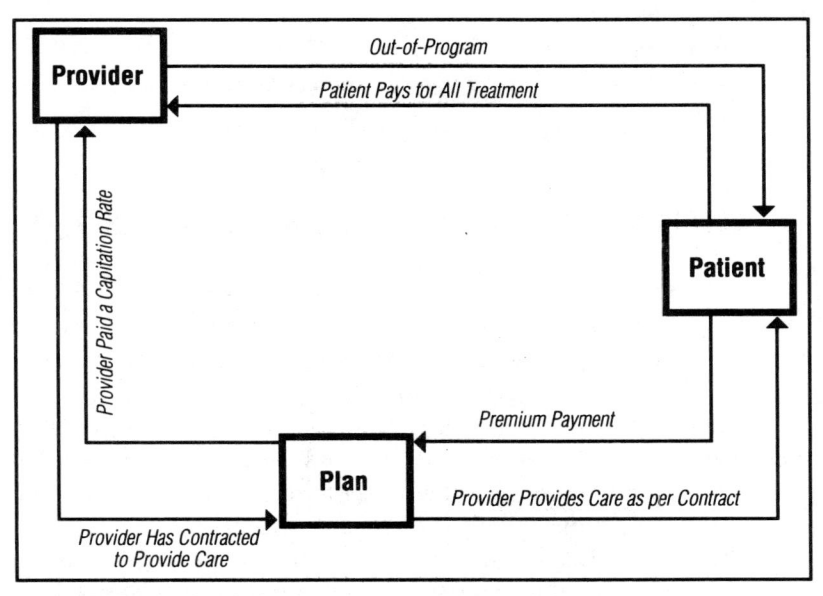

Figure 2–3. Capitation-based treatment systems

today, and this allows for managed-care dental plans to include attractive financial options for the dentist. These options can include:

- Volume purchasing of office supplies and professional equipment
- No-cost monitoring of OSHA compliance by the plan's quality assurance personnel
- "Hybrid" reimbursement programs that limit the captitated services, allowing the remainder of a stated scope of benefits to be reimbursed in a fee-for-service manner
- Special provider education courses and seminars

Opponents of capitated programs point out that a reduced scope of benefits may encourage dentists to "upsell" (convince patients to have higher cost, noncovered procedures performed) rather than deliver the least expensive, professionally ethical treatment. Opponents also point out that capitation programs tend towards underutilization of treatment, overutilization of specialty referrals, and do not allow the patient full freedom of choice in selecting a dentist from among all licensed providers in the service area.

Opponents also object to the placement of a dental provider "at-risk." Much of this opposition can be addressed with a more detailed explanation.

CAPITATION AND THE AT-RISK CONTRACT

An at-risk contract is one in which the provider is paid a flat fee per patient per month. Profitability comes from being able to manage the amount and type of care provided rather than from simply providing as much care as possible and billing for it.

Many dentists find it a difficult transition from a world where they are paid for performing treatments to a world where their compensation is no longer tied to production, but rather to their ability to manage the type and amount of therapy rendered to any single patient.

Placing a dental provider at-risk gives the purchaser some peace of mind that overutilization of services (overtreatment) will not be a factor in provider reimbursement, although undertreatment is still a possibility. Thus, there must be mechanisms in place that ensure the appropriateness of dental care rendered.

It is important for every dentist considering capitation-based managed-care contracts to know the various types of risk categories. There are many.

Utilization Risk

When determining what a reasonable capitation payment should be, the dental managed-care plan must share with the provider an accurate estimate of the amount of care that the covered population will require.

Price Risk

This is encountered when factors other than utilization increase your costs (office rent increases, salaries, etc.) relative to what it was anticipated the capitation amount would cover.

Adverse Selection Risk

This occurs when the population consists of a greater concentration of severe dental neglect than was originally estimated. Unlike utilization risk, this situation is not a function of the number of treatment visits required, but the high cost inherent to complete oral rehabilitation.

Demand Risk

If a given population of patients has never had access to a dentist before, and lacks "group experience," they may become high utilizers beyond a normal population's expected behavior.

Beta Risk

More of an actuarial term, this is when the number of assigned patients from the dental managed-care plan is too small to offset "outliers," or patients who consume lots of services. A dental provider is especially vulnerable to beta risk during his or her initial assignments of patients by the dental managed-care plan. During the weeks to months before an adequate patient capacity is reached, some plans allow fee-for-service billing to preclude this event. Others have predetermined monetary guarantees or "draws" against future payments.

Liability Risk

The provider must carefully evaluate the demographic content of the patient population for which he or she will be responsible. If these patients have a greater tendency to seek litigation against health-care providers, then the likelihood of a lawsuit has increased, and the reimbursement from the dental managed-care plan must reflect it.

Professional Risk

There is always a risk that associating with any organization may cause you to violate your professional ethics or have your professional reputation damaged. In *Wickline v. The State of California,* the courts firmly held that inadequate compensation did not allow a health-care provider to render substandard care. Dentists minimize professional risk by doing business only with those dental plans that present themselves with good track records and financial reserves.

DENTAL MAINTENANCE ORGANIZATIONS (DMOS)

Unfortunately, DMOs are often called by the terms "prepaid plan" or "capitation plan." This confuses the distinction between a form of provider payment and what amounts to an alternative dental-care delivery system. It is also an inaccurate depiction of dental managed-care plans' progress away from full capitation and towards more provider-friendly types of reimbursement.

DMOs often cover 100% of preventive and diagnostic services, including examinations, radiographs, cleanings, and fluoride applications (including sealants). Increasingly, patient co-payments are applied to the more costly primary and specialty care services, including fixed and removable prosthodontics and orthodontics. Annual or lifetime benefit ceilings are rarely a part of DMO limitations, much to the delight of patients and purchasers.

Point-of-Service Plans

A point-of-service plan is a hybrid plan that combines features of a DMO with a PPO. For those patients who remain within the DMO's

The Many Faces of Dental Plans

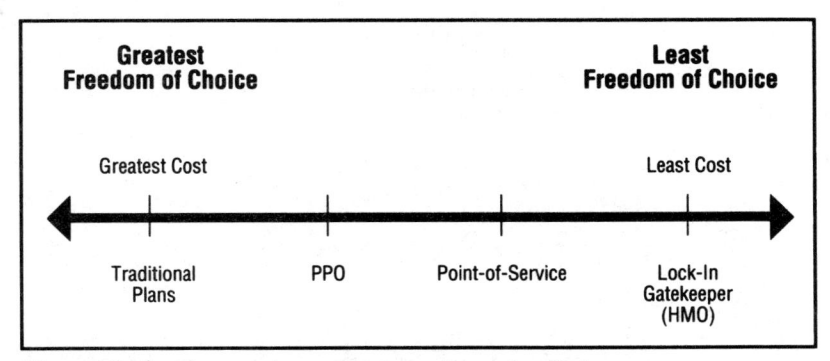

Figure 2–4. The spectrum of managed-care health insurance

provider network, higher benefits and lower (or zero) co-payments apply as opposed to those patients who select an outside provider.

The many faces of dental plans will add many more in the coming years. With the increasing popularity of managed medical-care plans, the adoption of managed-care principles and philosophies will fuel more hybridization, variation, and customization of dental-care delivery systems (see Fig. 2–4).

Chapter 3

Surviving Health Care Reform: Today and Beyond

"He had had much experience of physicians, and said, 'The only way to keep your health is to eat what you don't want, drink what you don't like, and do what you'd druther not.'"
Samuel Clemens (1835–1910), U.S. author. "Pudd'nhead Wilson's New Calendar," *Following the Equator*, (1897) from *The Columbia Dictionary of Quotations* (Columbia University Press, 1993).

Health-care reform is a national issue of immense proportions. The desire to reform the way our nation conducts health-care affairs, policies, and practices is really nothing new to the scene. Dr. Paul Elwood, currently of the Jackson Hole Group (a leading forum for health-care alternatives), was a strong advocate of national health-care reform as early as 1967. At that time, he spoke out against what he viewed as an increasingly fragmented health-care system in the United States.

Two years earlier, President Lyndon Johnson signed into legislation an amendment to the federal Social Security Act to create Medicaid and Medicare. While these programs have been invaluable towards increasing access to health care for millions of Americans, they and other programs have had great difficulties in controlling health-care costs. What has been seen as cost-control has primarily been cost-shifting. The federal government shifts certain responsibilities to the states; states attempt to either tighten eligibility guidelines or limit health benefits (along with reducing provider compensation); providers shift uncompensated costs or reduced income towards those patients with "better" insurance; the insurance companies and health plans raise premiums to offset the increased utilization of services and subsequent payouts; and the purchasers of health-care coverage (generally businesses) shift the increased costs towards their customers (see Fig. 3–1).

The arrival of the Clinton administration to the White House brought to the nation's attention the issue of health-care reform on a

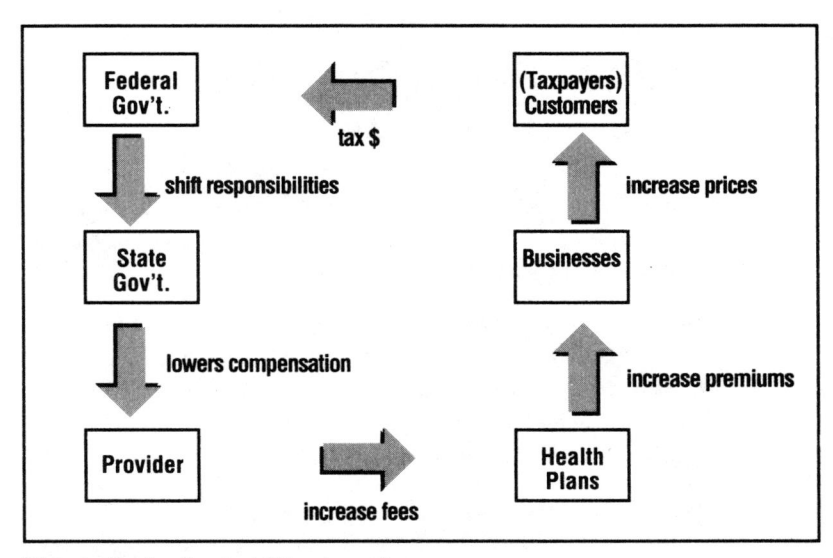

Figure 3–1. Cost-shifting paradigm

massive scale. The year 1993 will reside in the history books as having generated the greatest number of health-care reform proposals in American history. Consider the more notable efforts of that year:

- Clinton Health Security Plan (1993)
- Managed Competition Act of 1993 (Cooper & Grandy)
- The American Health Security Act of 1993 (McDermott)
- Health Equity and Access Reform Today Act of 1993 (Chafee)
- The Consumer Choice Health Security Act of 1993 (Nickles)
- Affordable Health Care Now Act of 1993 (Michel)

It is important to note that, regardless of the author, dentistry was generally either disregarded completely or relegated to a very minor role. This is disturbing, for while these reform acts may pass into oblivion, the manner in which dental benefits are handled in future versions may persist.

Since the Clinton Health Security Plan was so intensely scrutinized by Congress and the media, a review of its dental provisions is worthwhile.

CLINTON HEALTH SECURITY PLAN —HEALTH CARE ACT

According to the White House Domestic Policy Council's *The President's Health Security Plan*, (New York: Times Books, 1993) the dental care described in this section is the following:

> *(1) Emergency dental treatment, including simple extractions, for acute infections, bleeding, and injuries to natural teeth and oral structures for conditions requiring immediate attention to prevent risks to life or significant medical complications, as specified by the National Health Board.*
>
> *(2) Prevention and diagnosis of dental disease, including oral dental examinations, radiographs, dental sealants, fluoride application, and dental prophylaxis.*

(3) Treatment of dental disease, including routine fillings, prosthetics for genetic defects, periodontal maintenance, and endodontic services.

(4) Space maintenance procedures to prevent orthodontic complications.

(5) Interceptive orthodontic treatment to prevent severe malocclusion,

Coverage for dental care is subject to the following limitations:

(1) Prevention and diagnosis. Prior to January 1, 2001, the items and services described in subsection (a)(2) are covered only for individuals less than 18 years of age. On or after such date, such items and services are covered for all eligible individuals enrolled under a health plan, except that dental sealants are not covered for individuals 18 years of age or older.

(2) Treatment of dental disease. Prior to January 1, 2001, the items and services described in subsection (a)(3) are covered only for individuals less than 18 years of age. On or after such date, such items and services are covered for all eligible individuals enrolled under a health plan, except that orthodontic services are not covered for individuals 18 years of age or older.

(3) Space maintenance. The items and services described in subsection (a)(4) are covered only for individuals at least three years of age, but less than 13 years of age and

   (a) are limited to posterior teeth;

   (b) involved maintenance of a space or spaces for permanent posterior teeth that would otherwise be prevented from normal eruption if the space were not maintained; and

   (c) do not include a space maintainer that is placed within six months of the expected eruption of the permanent posterior tooth concerned.

(4) Interceptive orthodontic treatment. Prior to January 1, 2001, the items and services described in subsection (a)(5) are not covered. On or after such date, such items and services are

covered only for individuals at least six years of age, but less than 12 years of age.

Therein lies the entire scope of benefits, including limitations, of dental care for Americans in the president's formal health plan. In the president's speech to the Joint Session of Congress, **there was not a single mention of dentistry or dental services.** To find any mention of dentistry again, one had to wait for "Health Security—The President's Report to the American People."

During this 1993 report, the president had only this to say about dental benefits: "Beginning in the year 2001, the nationally guaranteed benefits package will expand to include the following: . . . preventive dental care for adults . . . orthodontia if necessary to prevent reconstructive surgery for children."

The dental benefits for adults are meager, to say the least. The benefits for children are more substantial, given the stated limitations, but strangely follow those already established in most states providing children's dental services under Medicaid eligible populations. For those children who reside in families not eligible for Medicaid, the federal Early and Periodic Screening, Diagnosis, and Treatment program (EPSDT) generally provides all medically necessary dental services for families earning up to 200% of the federally established poverty level.

It is interesting to note that, if the federal government chose to do so, by merely increasing the federal poverty level benchmark they could theoretically close the gap between covered and noncovered children populations for dental care. Such an action would sidestep the need for sweeping reform legislation, but would be just another example of the federal government shifting responsibilities towards the states.

For the adult dental patient with a traditional fee-for-service program, there is real danger in what any future health-care reform may portend. Two well-organized responses to the issue of dentistry and national health-care reform are worthy of note. The first was by the American Dental Association. The second was spearheaded by Delta Dental Plans, who called their group "The Dental Health Coalition."

AMERICAN DENTAL ASSOCIATION— "HEALTH CARE THAT WORKS"

On March 6, 1994, a group of more than 300 dentists representing the ADA descended on lawmakers and canvassed Capitol Hill. The message was blunt—leave dentistry out of health-care reform. Three main points were made by the dentist-lobbyists:

- Dental benefits should remain tax deductible
- Federal funds should be directed to persons with the greatest financial need and least access to dental care
- Dental care need not be covered in a basic benefit package since the dental care system already embraces the goals of reformers

In reviewing the health-care position paper 42H-1993 put forth by the ADA's House of Delegates several months earlier, one can see the stance more clearly; their goal is to

> *maintain the advantages of the current dental care and dental benefits system, which would not require inclusion of dental benefits for groups currently receiving regular dental care, and which would not require public sector participation and subsequent cost transfer. The Association strongly opposes any change in the tax deductibility of current dental benefit coverage.*
>
> *The Association supports the opportunity for (a) small employers to purchase dental plans in the private sector, or (b) development of cooperative dental-benefit purchasing alliances administered in the private sector, which will provide fee-for-service dental care as a preferred option.*[12]

The message being sent out to Congress from the House of Delegates essentially says:

1. Leave dentistry out of health-care reform

2. Do not establish universal care or an "all-payer" system that would displace those patients already in "good" dental plans

3. Health-care purchasing alliances are supported as long as fee-for-service remains the preferred option

It is not expected that the American Dental Association will modify this position any time in the near future.

THE DENTAL HEALTH COALITION

The Dental Health Coalition consists of a group of California dental, business, labor, and health-benefit organizations. At a press conference on April 5, 1994, in Sacramento, the coalition called for a health plan with comprehensive dental benefits for all Americans. In concert with the ADA, the coalition opposed the taxation of dental benefits under health-care reform.

The American Dental Association did not join this coalition, nor did the California Dental Association. In fact, both organizations have been rather vocal about their opposition to the coalition's main message to Congress. Dr. John Zapp, Executive Director of the ADA, had this to say: "Once you start down that track to be included across the board in a program that is going to require any type of federal resources or subsidies, you automatically lose the tax deductibility because that is how the government is going to fund (health care) reform."[13] Going even further, Dr. Zapp stated that "dentists need to remember that because Delta is not a dental organization, we shouldn't expect them to have the same objectives that dentists do."[14]

These views, one by organized dentistry and the other by a coalition dominated by the dental benefit plan industry, are not surprisingly disparate. While both groups realize that all dental benefit programs would suffer if tax deductibility was lost, the dental benefit industry wants to be a part of health-care reform, and organized dentistry does not.

Because the tax deductibility of supplemental benefits (including dental) beyond a standard benefits package would be eliminated, employers are faced with a dilemma. Dental benefits for their employees could be eliminated altogether, or the benefit could be retained (at a much higher cost) as a negotiating point during collective bargaining.

Flexible spending accounts, which have grown in popularity among workers and benefit managers, would be eliminated under many health-care reform plans. Since such accounts are not taxed presently, such an action would amount to an ersatz tax increase.

Given the totality of all of these aforementioned effects on employee dental benefits, it is quite possible that if health-care reform results in higher costs (including taxes) to those employers whose employees already enjoy dental benefits, they may gravitate towards managed-care dental plans as a cost-saving option.

SHOULD DENTAL BENEFITS EVEN BE A PART OF HEALTH CARE REFORM?

In looking beyond any transient attempts at health-care reform, dentists must consider what the future will bring. We have seen substantial evidence that:

1. Dental benefits will be of a lower priority than medical concerns

2. Taxation of dental benefits will be an ongoing debate in political circles

3. Professional dental organizations and dental benefit plans have taken opposite positions on key points

It seems impossible to argue that dentistry should not be considered a part of the core benefits of any health-care plan, whether it comes from Capitol Hill or an executive boardroom. Such a position places dentistry as a profession whose impact on the total health of Americans is negligible—a ridiculous idea, as well as a dangerous one to plant into the minds of politicians and bureaucrats.

Leaving dentistry out of any reform package is to ignore the following facts:

- Oral disease affects the majority of Americans

- Dental disease is not self-limiting, nor are the effects reversible by patient actions alone in all cases except gingivitis and incipient caries

- Sixty percent of Americans are without any dental plan coverage of any kind

- Increases in dental fees still outpace inflation

- Exclusion of dental benefits from any core benefit package will reduce accessibility to care if tax exclusion is lost (since taxable benefits will help to pay for any health-care reform package)

WHAT TYPES OF DENTAL SERVICES SHOULD BE INCLUDED IN A CORE OF HEALTH BENEFITS?

In order to hold down the costs of dental benefits, a national health-care package will most likely include the following as the dental portion of any core of health benefits:

- Diagnostic and preventive services
- Basic restorative services (mainly "fillings," although the ADA defines these services as part of preventive measures)
- Periodontal scaling and root planing (including maintenance)
- Pulpal therapy on deciduous teeth
- Limited exodontia
- Emergency care

Note that these dental benefits fit nicely into a dental managed-care delivery system and would appear too "limited" for a viable indemnity-based program. This is why any future national health-care reform plan that includes dental benefits in the core package will not support fee-for-service reimbursement of dentists. Managed-care will be embraced for any and all health-care services that make the "cut."

If dental benefits do not make it into the core package, then all signs point to the loss of tax-free dental benefits, whereby purchasers will look towards dental managed care to make up for lessened purchasing power. Purchasers will also find that full-service health plans, with medical and dental fully integrated into one delivery system, will start to predominate in a free-market system. Medical plans will consolidate with dental plans, decreasing the administrative burden of two companies, and allowing purchasers of health benefits the advantage of dealing only with a few comprehensive health plans.

STRATEGIES FOR THE FUTURE

- Economies of scale will prevail—dentists should start considering group practices, IPA structures (discussed later), and other methods of consolidation.
- Analyze all managed-care opportunities—discard the poorly designed plans, but strive to become a provider in at least one acceptable dental managed-care network.
- Members of organized dental groups should demand that such groups be realistic and responsive to the future of dental managed care in national health-care reform.
- Minority-group dentists, often the mainstream providers for their own ethnic and cultural groups, should demand greater representation in organized dentistry and special consideration during the national transition towards dental managed care.

No one has a clear view into the future of health-care reform. To the astute dental practitioner, the lessons learned from the various attempts at national health-care reform will be a call to action and not the sounding of retreat.

Chapter 4

What Is Managed Care in Dentistry?

> *"In the greatest confusion there is still an open channel to the soul. It may be difficult to find because by mid-life it is overgrown, and some of the wildest thickets that surround it grow out of what we describe as our education. But the channel is always there, and it is our business to keep it open, to have access to the deepest part of ourselves."*
> Saul Bellow (1915–), U.S. novelist.
> Foreword to *The Closing of the American Mind* by Allan Bloom, (1987).

Unfortunately, managed care is not copyrighted or trademarked. Any dental plan can call itself "managed care," even if what is actually "managed" is but the tiniest portion of their dental programs. Most dentists still refer to these as capitation programs, and even at that the participation levels are increasing (see Fig. 4–1).

With this in mind, some organizations have decided to define managed care as a process, with objectives (or outcomes) in mind. The state of Hawaii's QUEST program for Medicaid dental patients defines it:

> *Under the existing fee-for-service methodology, providers are paid based on established reimbursement rates for the services provided. There is little incentive for the providers to manage the utilization of health services by the recipient because provider reimbursement is not linked to prudent usage of health-care resources by the recipients.*
>
> *Managed care is being introduced to meet the following objectives:*

- Cost containment
- Provision of appropriate care
- Increased access to quality care
- Improved health status of the recipients

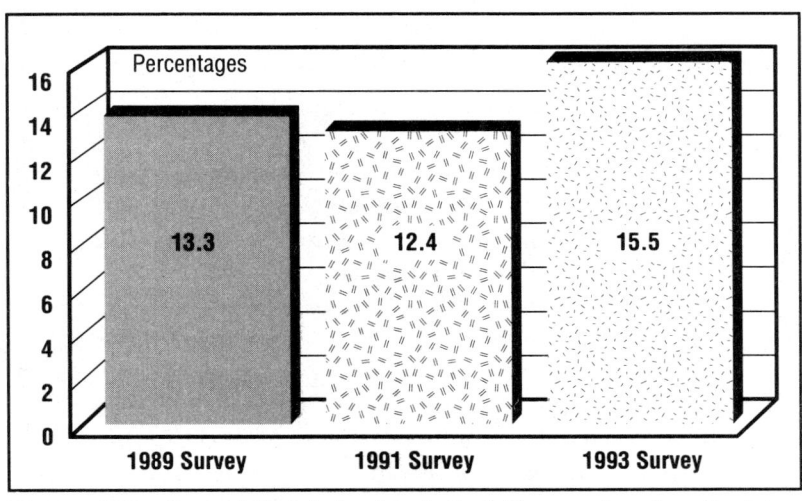

Figure 4–1. Prepaid dental plan (capitation) (Source: American Dental Association, 1994)

> *Managed care is a method of health-care delivery that integrates the financing, administration, and delivery of health services. Managed care is a coordinated delivery system made up of pre-established networks of health-care providers providing a defined package of benefits under pre-established reimbursement rates. The concepts of managed care include:*
>
> Improving access, ensuring appropriate utilization of services and enhancing recipient and provider satisfaction. *Case managers are used to coordinate the care of the recipient and refer the recipient to specialists and other services as directed by the primary care dentist (PCD).*
>
> Controlling costs while maintaining quality of care. *Quality of care means furnishing safe dental care within established dental standards. Measures of assessing quality of care include provider credentialing, performance monitoring, utilization management, and follow-up with corrective action as needed. Cost-control measures include preadmission certification, prior authorization, utilization reviews, and case management.*[15]

The one put forth by the California Department of Health Services is more generalized:

> *Managed care, broadly stated, is a planned, comprehensive approach to the provision of quality health care that combines clinical services and administrative procedures within an integrated, coordinated system that is carefully constructed to provide timely access to primary care and other necessary services in a cost-effective manner. . . . In addition, quality of care can better be assured in managed-care systems than in fee-for-service. Unlike fee-for-service, providers operating in a managed-care environment are formally and systematically linked in a manner that allows quality*

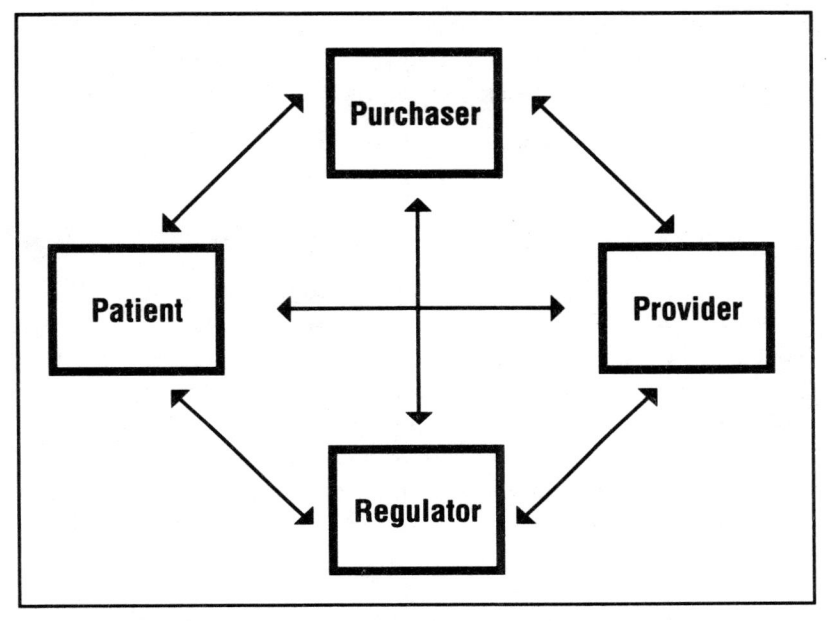

Figure 4–2. Managed care provides linkages

of care to be rationally assessed and accountability for care to be established and monitored (see Fig. 4–2).[16]

The Health Insurance Association of America in 1990 defined managed care as an integrated health-care financing and delivery system that covers persons through:

1. arrangements with selected providers to furnish comprehensive services to members,
2. explicit standards for selecting providers,
3. formal, ongoing quality assurance and utilization review programs, and
4. financial incentives for members to use plan providers and procedures.

The American Dental Association puts forth a terse, and definitely biased, definition of managed care as a "cost-containment system that directs the utilization of health benefits by:

a. restricting the type, level, and frequency of treatment,

b. limiting the access to care, and

c. controlling the level of reimbursement for services."[17]

The dentist who is facing managed care for the first time is likely to see all of these definitions put forth at some point in time, or perhaps none at all. In reality, managed care is a process. This process is defined by its elements. What dental plans should be telling you is not so much that they **are** managed care but **to what degree** they are managed care.

There exists a triad—three essential elements, broad in scope—that no managed-care program can fail to address: access, quality of care, and cost containment.

ACCESS

Most dentists, acutely aware of the national debate raging over health-care reform, would naturally assume that the containment of health-care costs would be the primary factor in managed care. Actually, of the three essential elements that make up the triad, it is the accessibility to services that pulls rank above the other two elements.

Consider this: A dental program is established with a liberal scope of benefits and places minimal financial burden on the backs of patients. Furthermore, the premium structure is such that purchasers of health plans consider it a best buy. Sounds great so far, with one notable exception: there is virtually no access to dental services for the patients. Perhaps the plan failed to attract sufficient numbers of providers; the reimbursement was inadequate; those providers who did sign on with the plan had no additional capacity in their practices for any of these patients; or a large clinic setting (or "staff-model" office) was established too distant from the residence or workplace for most patients. Even cultural and linguistic differences between dentists and patients can create invisible barriers to the accessibility of care.

Moving from the hypothetical to the real world, consider the famous *Clark v. Coye* federal court decision against the California Medicaid dental program, better known as Denti-Cal. Key to the judge's decision was that while the dental program had an adequate scope of benefits, it lacked adequate patient access to those benefits. The plaintiffs prevailed, and program costs for the state of California were projected to eclipse $800 million by the year 1995.

A number of factors operate under the auspices of access and deserve individual explanation.

SERVICE AREA

A plan must establish a distinct, geographical area within which its dental program will operate. This "service area" might encompass the entire United States or be restricted to within certain metropolitan city limits. Within this area, time and distance standards must be established and enforced. For those dental plans licensed by the California Department of Corporations under the Knox-Keene Act of 1975, patients should be able to travel no more than 15 miles or 30 minutes to a participating dental office. In addition, time-specific appointments in response to a patient's initial request for routine or specialty nonemergency care should be available within two weeks. Many plans accomplish this with sophisticated computer programs that show detailed maps by zip code. Provider locations and patient locations can be matched accurately.

EMERGENCY SERVICES

One of the driving forces behind the medical models of managed care is misutilization of hospital services during emergencies. Many patients were using their local hospital's emergency room as an "after-hours clinic" for problems that could have been resolved in a doctor's office.

For dentists, managed care will require that the plan provide for 24-hour, seven-days-a-week access to emergency care. Some programs place this burden squarely on the backs of the dentist; others have arrangements with central facilities to handle all after-hour problems; still others place their providers on a rotational on-call status.

Such policies are fine if the patient is still within the dental managed-care plan's service area, but what if he or she is not? Dental plans must have policies to cover dental emergencies that occur outside of the plan's service area. This is generally the only instance where a dental managed-care enrollee is allowed to receive dental treatment from outside providers—and then such treatment is limited to emergency services only. These providers may call the plan's phone number to receive information on reimbursement—others require the patient to pay for the services, and the dental managed-care plan will reimburse the patient with a proper receipt and documentation of the emergency condition.

LINGUISTIC AND CULTURAL SENSITIVITIES

It is not uncommon for a member of an ethnic group to seek out health care from providers of his or her own ethnicity. Language barriers are usually nonexistent, and unique cultural qualities that may affect a patient's approach to health care can be accommodated easily. Since established dental plans pay close attention to service area demographics anyway, their managed-care products have no excuse for ignoring these factors.

It would be wise for the dentist whose practice is predominately oriented towards an ethnic group, or who is part of an active dental organization (i.e., Korean Dentists of the USA, Indian Dental Association of California) that represents an ethnic group to ensure that participation in a plan's provider network would not interfere with these relationships.

PROVIDER NETWORK

The ideal managed-care plan would systematically link all of its providers in such a way that a de facto partnership develops. Within a service area, a plan would seek out providers in forming a network—one that would incorporate all of the factors noted previously, as well as meet any special needs of the patients and purchasers.

This is an extremely tall order. When dealing with traditional fee-for-service plans, dentists were not assigned patients, put at-risk for their dental needs, nor required to participate (to any real degree) with quality assurance and utilization review functions. Plans were busy with claims processing and marketing functions. Not only have the priorities changed for both groups, but the need to establish a viable provider network implies the need for first-class communication between both groups.

The mistakes made during establishment of provider networks during the early attempts at dental managed care are partly to blame for today's fear of it. Many insurance companies and dental service organizations simply approached those dentists who, from their filed fees and computer-based practice profiles, already charged less for dental services than other dentists in a specific service area. Through the use of complicated contractual encumbrances on these dentists ("hold harmless" clauses and the like), early managed care was really just a capitated dental program. Dentists suffered from adverse selection, low capitation fees, and other ills inherent to poor plan administration.

Managed care in dentistry cannot meet its prime goal of access when its provider network is inferior. This does not mean to imply inferior dentists or inferior dentistry. Plans must realize that maintaining excellent provider networks requires a dedicated effort from both dentists and the plan itself.

Chapter 7 is devoted to dealing with this sensitive and multifaceted issue of provider networks.

REFERRAL SYSTEM

Many providers, at first glance, will find this portion of dental managed care to be very intrusive. The primary care dentist-to-specialist relationship is a sacred one to many dentists. A sizable number will argue against a plan that has not enrolled one of "their" referral specialists, saying that the courts often hold the referring dentist partly responsible for any substandard care rendered by the specialist.

In dental managed care, all providers are subject to a credentialing process and subsequently privileged to render a certain range of services within the plan's scope of benefits. Since managed-care plans are legally on the hook for the actions of their provider network, this fear is unjustified.

The primary care dentist (PCD) acts as a gatekeeper for any

specialty care. The gatekeeper concept is more crucial to medical managed care than dental managed care for several reasons:

- Medical patients tend to self-refer directly to specialists.
- Medical patients often lack a primary care physician with whom the specialist can coordinate care, leading to incomplete case management.
- Medical specialists (whose numbers are about 70–80% of the entire population of physicians in the nation) often perform procedures that a primary care physician could perform at a lower fee.

Nevertheless, the gatekeeper concept is an important one for dentistry, too. It is the PCD who:

- Determines if referral to a specialist is necessary
- Coordinates treatment with that specialist so that primary and preventive care is not disrupted while specialty care continues
- Provides continuity of care by keeping the master dental record and ensuring that patients do not become "lost" during the course of complex treatment plans and multiple referral patterns

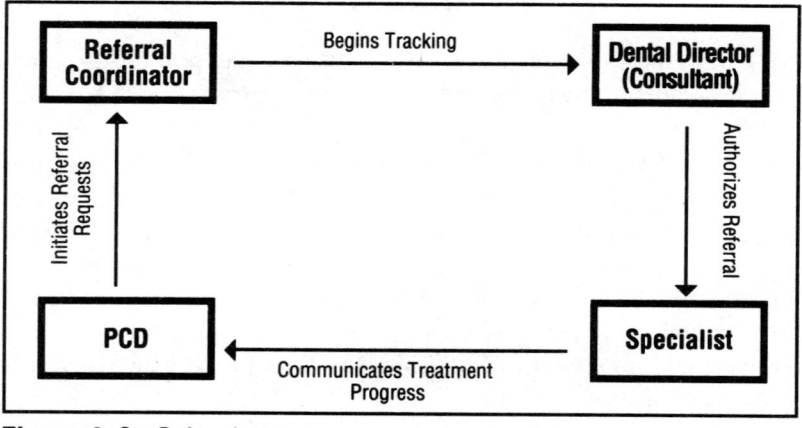

Figure 4–3. Referral system

It is incumbent upon the plan to provide an adequate tracking and monitoring system for all referrals (see Fig. 4–3). Usually, the plan's dental director will review certain types of referrals for dental necessity. Additionally, referral patterns of a particular PCD may indicate overutilization or underutilization of specialty care.

The dental managed-care plan must also ensure that their referral systems to not place unreasonable constraints upon their primary care dentists. Dental managed-care plans must ensure that:

- Adequate numbers and types of specialists are available to their PCDs
- Referral policies do not impose an arbitrary number of attempted dental treatment visits by the PCD as a condition prior to the PCD initiating any specialty referral request
- All referral requests are processed in a timely manner
- Authorization of any reasonable and appropriate referral request will not result in the imposition of any financial penalty or disincentive to the PCD

QUALITY ASSURANCE PROGRAM

Businesses in America are no strangers to quality assurance programs. Great strides have been made in this area, starting with programs such as Total Quality Management (TQM), Continuous Quality Improvement (CQI), and a host of other off-the-shelf programs.

In dentistry, we have been trained in dental school to be hypercritical with judging the technical aspects of our profession. This leads to a constricted view of quality—mention the word to most dentists, and they will tell you about marginal integrity, restoration longevity, and similar clinically related aspects to dental procedures. These statements reflect technical quality, which is but a subset of a patient's entire quality of care.

Managed-care programs should have an ongoing quality assurance program that contains the following elements:

- Quality of care assessments

- Utilization review
- Peer review (see Fig. 4-4)
- Patient (member) grievance review
- Provider grievance review
- Case management review
- Continuity of care standards
- Dental record standards
- Environmental health and safety/infection control

Dear Dr. Quattlebaum:

Enclosed are the chart and radiographs of Roxanne Martin, the patient about whom I spoke with Lisa on March 5. The patient has complained that the DMO dentist whom she originally selected gave her a 10-minute rubber-cup prophylaxis and scaled only four lower teeth. She has always had a hygienist perform her cleanings in the past and says she has never had her teeth cleaned in less than 45 minutes.

As a member of the peer review committee, I would appreciate it if you would arrange a screening appointment for Ms. Martin. The DMO peer review forms are enclosed, including a note from our grievance coordinator.

Please send the bill for this examination to my attention for payment. If you feel that Ms. Martin needs immediate attention, give me a call.

Thank you and the other peer review members for helping.

Sincerely,

M.C. Progressive, D.D.S.
Dental Director
DMO

Figure 4-4. Sample peer review request letter

Obviously, a quality assurance program could be assembled with all of the components listed here and people might not know what to do with them. Luckily, there exists a myriad of associations and government agencies that have made the "translation" of generic QA programs into ones useful in the health-care arena. They include guidelines issued by the following:

- Health Care Financing Administration
- National Committee on Quality Assurance
- American Board of Quality Assurance and Utilization Review Physicians
- California Dental Association
- California Department of Corporations

The discussion of how a quality-oriented dental managed-care plan utilizes its QAP is reserved for Chapter 5.

COST CONTAINMENT

There must be a fine balance between prudent financial practices and optimal patient outcomes. In health care, this balance is finer than in any other industry. The courts have made it quite clear that the preservation of human life is priority one—this is why no hospital may refuse an emergency patient that has not been medically stabilized.

For dentists, patient morbidity is not of constant concern. The use of inferior supplies in a dental practice, however, is a concern. Most dentists would not mind using a less-expensive impression material if the clinical results were not compromised. Minor deviations from government-mandated infection control practices are tempting to even the most ethical dentist. The ideal treatment outcome is often patient satisfaction—not always an easy accomplishment in the real world of dental practice.

Dentistry will be practically immune to the effects of health-care rationing. The current oversupply of dentists, the lower costs of dental care versus medical treatments, and the fact that many dental procedures are discretionary—these factors and more point out that the actual denial of treatment for a life-threatening dental condition is remote.

The real pressures brought on by cost containment will center more on dental practice environment than actual dental procedures. As Dr. Max Schoen points out, large group practices have a built-in economy of scale that will place them in a more competitive position than the solo dental practitioner.

Dental managed-care plans are finding themselves squeezed by the pressures of the free market to develop more efficient ways of administering their programs. Individual dentists will be forced to become efficient practice managers as well as case managers of patients in order to remain competitive (and thereby attractive) to managed-care companies.

Now that you have had your "primer" in dental managed care, you will be more comfortable as we expand our discussion of the previous topics (and blend in new ones) in the chapters ahead.

Chapter 5

Quality Assurance and Dental Managed Care

"What I call a good patient is one who, having found a good physician, sticks to him till he dies."

Oliver Wendell Holmes, Sr. (1809–94),
U.S. writer, physician. Lecture,
2 March 1871, New York.

The dentist who desires to participate in dental managed care will also be participating in quality assurance programs (QAPs). Each of the dental managed-care plans will have QAPs, and dentists who are part of their provider networks will be contractually obligated to participate in them. The dentist's first introduction to dental managed care's quality assurance programs will most likely be the preenrollment process one must complete before entering a provider network. We will leave that discussion for another chapter.

What initially may seem burdensome should be looked at as a

unique opportunity. QAPs in industry and medicine have progressed to the point where, when properly managed by the dental plan, intrusion is supplanted by education. The managed-care provider learns from an exchange of ideas facilitated by the QAP. This is a giant leap that fee-for-service plans have been unable to make, even though they talk about quality. The following is an excerpt from a newsletter sent out by Delta Dental Plan of New Jersey: "Service corporations, like Delta, have another concern when it comes to new procedures. Technically, service corporations are contracted to provide services through participating dentists. Compare this with insurance companies, which simply reimburse patients for the cost of services. Sometimes this is a subtle distinction, but it is an important one because it means that the service corporation must be able to *guarantee the quality and longevity of covered services.*"[18] If dental service corporations, such as Delta, were literally guaranteeing the quality of dental care delivered by their participating dentists, dental managed care would not be as attractive to purchasers.

Other industries besides health-care industries have developed standards such as ANSI/ASQC Standard A# (1987) which defines quality assurance as "all those planned or systematic actions necessary to provide confidence that a product or service will satisfy given needs."[19]

The managed-care provider need not worry that he will face a QAP intended for one industry that has been forced into a managed-care mold. In fact, there are five distinct and accomplished national managed-care accrediting bodies that have already completed the translation of QAP into the health professions. They are:

- National Committee for Quality Assurance
- American Accreditation Program, Inc.
- Utilization Review Accreditation Commission
- Joint Commission on Accreditation of Healthcare Organizations
- Accreditation Association for Ambulatory Health Care

For those health professionals who find themselves in career positions with managed-care plans and desire internationally recognized board certification, the American Board of Quality Assurance and Utilization Review Physicians exists for this purpose. Any allied health

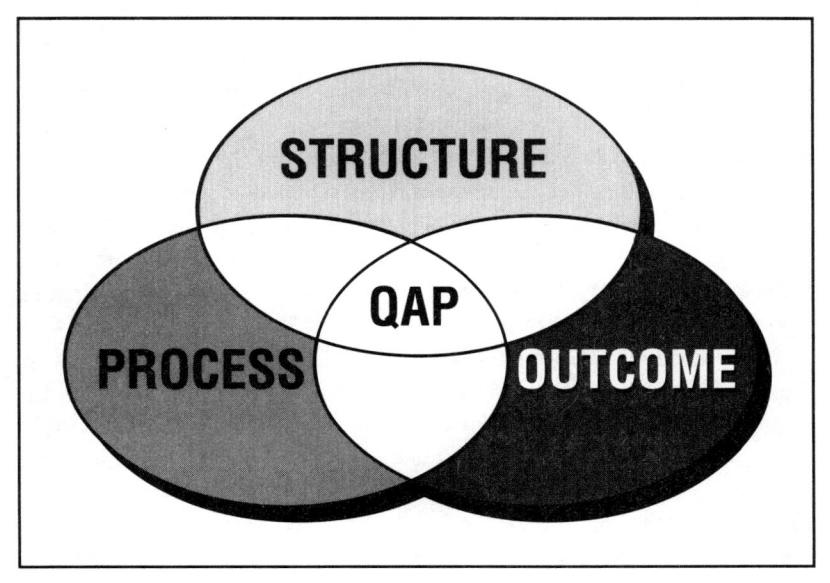

Figure 5–1. The triad of QAP

professionals may seek board certification from this organization, whose examination and certification process is conducted by the National Board of Medical Examiners.

All QAPs orient themselves around a basic triad of structure, process, and outcome (see Fig. 5–1).

Structure. This element is concerned with the physical items necessary for patient care. For the provider, this will deal with such things as: office capacity for patients, central sterilization areas, OSHA compliance, waiting-room capacity, and other tangibles.

Process. This element is concerned with how the patient actually receives care—the quality of the care, appropriateness of treatment decisions, case management, and even cultural and linguistic concerns that may alter treatment decisions.

Outcome. This element concerns itself with the outcome of patient care. Put very simply, Is the patient better or worse as the result of having received dental treatment?

Much progress has been made in medical circles with outcomes studies as an important measurement of quality. The use of outcomes studies is somewhat compromised in dentistry at the present time. In medicine, the patient's diagnosis is noted with International Classification of Diseases (ICD-9) codes, and the treatment process is tracked from that origin. As a result, medical outcomes studies are readily correlated to the patient's original diagnosis. The question of whether a patient became better or worse can be answered more completely. Indeed, medical HMOs have developed many measures to assist their QAPs (see Fig. 5–2).

In the dental profession, although ICD-9 codes do exist for most dental pathoses, dental schools do not teach us to use them, and the dental benefits industry has driven claims processing with the use of ADA procedure codes. This poses a serious problem for outcomes studies, as there is no diagnostic focal point available unless one can be generated from patient records or an actual patient-screening examination performed retrospective to the treatment received.

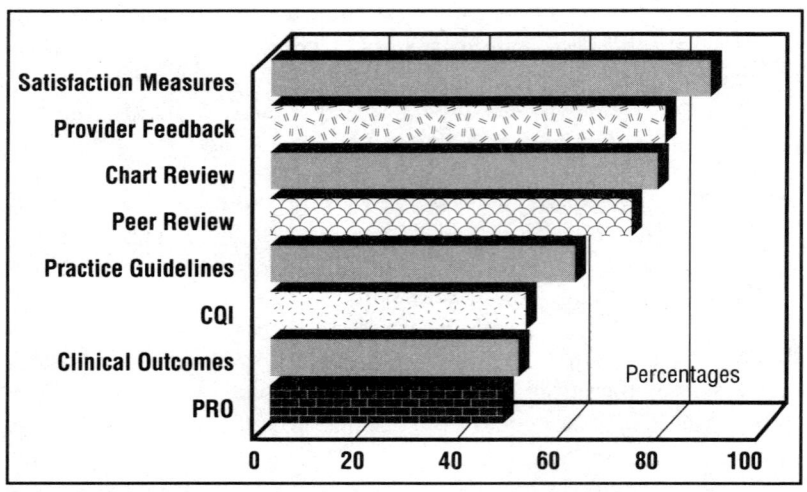

Figure 5–2. Medical HMO quality control measures [Source: The Interstudy Competitive Edge (Group Health Insurance Association of America, 1991)]

COMPONENTS OF A DENTAL QUALITY ASSURANCE PROGRAM

In dental managed care, the QAP will be heavily relied upon, not just to monitor dental care, but to assure that the full assimilation of quality goals has been met throughout the dental plan. This is a tall order, and most dental plans will identify separate components to their QAP. The following are deemed basic components of a QAP, though many managed-care plans elect to incorporate more (a more inclusive list is found in Chapter 4):

- Peer review
- Utilization review
- Patient and provider grievances
- OSHA compliance/infection control
- Case management

These may all reside under a central QAP committee (for large dental managed-care plans) or be separate subcommittees that directly report to a central QAP committee. Regardless of where these components would reside on an organization chart, they merit individual explanations.

PEER REVIEW

As has already been established by professional organizations such as the American Dental Association and the California Dental Association, dentists are the best judges of other dentists in terms of treatment quality, appropriateness, dental record maintenance, etc. Much of what is used by existing dental managed-care plans is based on peer-review protocols already in use by the profession.

What dental plans will have to become more cognizant of are the constraints and directives established in the Health Care Quality Improvement Act of 1986. The act is noted for its creation of the National Practitioner Data Bank—a repository of information concerning the performance of health professionals in the course of their duties. The act is explicit in those details, found mostly through peer-review processes, that must be reported to the data bank.

The information contained within the National Practitioner Data Bank cannot be seen by just anyone—but the bank can be queried by managed-care plans in their selection process for provider networks and professional staffing. Dentists should start getting in the habit of querying the data bank on a regular basis, or whenever a peer review committee has taken action concerning their practice activities. The National Practitioner Data Bank was not intended to destroy careers, but information can be misreported or misapplied, with serious consequences if not readily corrected.

UTILIZATION REVIEW

Every dental plan in existence currently maintains some sort of utilization review (or utilization management). In fact, how a dental plan conducts its review of participating providers and their billing practices is considered proprietary information and is jealously guarded by most plans. The more effective the utilization management, the more competitive the dental plan will be in the hostile marketplace.

Utilization review in the fee-for-service environment focuses almost exclusively on cost controls. It is entirely retrospective in nature, since patients have already received the billed dental treatment. With complicated computer programs, well-trained paraprofessional auditors and dental consultants, an astute dental plan can tell much about how any specific dentist practices dentistry. Consider the information that is usually submitted in a claims process:

- Patient radiographs
- Procedure codes
- Narrative documentation

Given a long history of claims paid to a population of providers, dental plans are able to develop practice profiles for each dentist. Dentists who bill for too many root canals, for example, would be identified as outliers in comparison to the usual billing patterns of their colleagues. Outliers can trigger formal audits by the dental plan, and this is one way in which the appropriateness of care can be measured. Unfortunately, though billing patterns may help a dental plan in controlling costs, retrospective reviews are generally blind to the other measures of modern quality assurance.

In dental managed care, policies and procedures in utilization review will augment the evaluation of dental care in others areas of the QAP. Mechanisms will detect the underutilization of dental services as well as the overutilization of them. Aggregate data will establish practice patterns, conduct trend analysis, and develop statistical profiles in prospective and concurrent modes, not just retrospectively.

Instead of data collection being solely derived from claims processing, the managed-care dentist will use "encounter data reporting," with each visit by a patient being one encounter. This reporting requirement can be as simple as checking off the correct boxes on an encounter form, reflecting what procedures were done for each patient. A single form can also tell the dental plans if broken appointments or no-shows are being abused by a patient. More importantly, encounter data reporting lends itself ideally to electronic data submission, since no other documentation (i.e., radiographs) must follow the electronic facsimile in a separate mailing through the U.S. postal system.

Dentists generally find that encounter data reporting in managed care is much simpler and less intrusive than complicated claim forms, radiograph submission requirements, complex documentation requests, and preauthorization of benefits, all of which are ubiquitous to fee-for-service plans.

PATIENT AND PROVIDER GRIEVANCES

All grievances and complaints, regardless of origin, that relate to possibly inadequate quality of care, poor treatment decisions, or even provider misconduct will first come to the attention of the managed-care plan's dental director. The director's investigation and recommendations, assisted by the plan's grievance coordinator, are then routed to the QAP committee for final action.

Nondental-related grievances or complaints are logged and tracked, and it is then the responsibility of the grievance coordinator to make full reports to the QAP. Problems reported by members are generally handled separately from those coming from providers.

The process of handling complaints is certainly not new territory for fee-for-service dental plans. The scope and final resolution of grievances is far greater in dental managed care due to the demands of the QAP. Satisfaction with the dental managed-care plan must be established with patients, purchasers, providers, and government regulators. Patient satisfaction surveys are heavily used by nearly all dental managed-care plans, provide valuable feedback to the dental plan, and are an excellent marketing tool.

OSHA COMPLIANCE/INFECTION CONTROL

For every dentist who has had to deal with the ever-increasing demands of OSHA and CDC guidelines, dental managed care should offer substantial relief. Preenrollment audits of dental offices prior to participation in a network are intended to educate and correct facility deficiencies, notably in this area. Some dental managed-care plans already offer specially trained personnel to help identify shortcomings and develop the appropriate corrective action plan (CAP) that will resolve infection control problems. All CAPs are reviewed by the QAP committee which can alert a plan to problems within its network (and a need for increased provider education efforts) while the problem is still in its infancy.

CASE MANAGEMENT

Case management principles are taught in every American dental school. The purpose of the QAP is to ensure that the primary care dentist carries out this responsibility, which includes:

- Determination of oral-health risk
- Identification of oral disease (diagnosis)
- Development of a complete treatment plan

- Consultation and referral to dental specialists (where needed)
- Follow-up care and maintenance recall schedules

Parameters of care come into play here, for they greatly assist the PCD in making appropriate decisions. A number of specialty groups have already established formal parameters of care within their respective fields, including:

- American Association of Endodontics
- American Academy of Pediatric Dentistry
- American Academy of Oral & Maxillofacial Surgery

When the remainder of the dental profession follows their lead, the work of QAPs will become stronger and more directed towards favorable outcomes.

Much progress has been performed in the art and science of quality assurance. From the phenomenal turnaround of post-World War II Japanese industry (largely credited to W. Edwards Deming, an American) to the current work of Philip Crosby (proponent of "zero defects") and others, quality assurance programs are constantly improving. Dental managed care will benefit from this evolution, but more importantly, so will the managed-care dentist.

CHAPTER 6

ENCOUNTER DATA REPORTING— A FAREWELL TO CLAIMS

> *"It seems to me that there must be an ecological limit to the number of paper pushers the earth can sustain, and that human civilization will collapse when the number of, say, tax lawyers exceeds the world's total population of farmers, weavers, fisherpersons, and pediatric nurses."*
>
> BARBARA EHRENREICH (1941–), U.S. AUTHOR, COLUMNIST. "PREMATURE PRAGMATISM," *THE WORST YEARS OF OUR LIVES* (1991) FROM *THE COLUMBIA DICTIONARY OF QUOTATIONS* (COLUMBIA UNIVERSITY PRESS, 1993).

The U.S. health-care system has the highest proportion of administrative costs in the world. Our pluralistic health insurance woes are not confined to medical benefit plans alone. Dental plans suffer from variable payment rates, dozens of separate utilization review systems, complex eligibility standards, and high marketing costs.

It is estimated that as much as 10% of the nation's $940 billion health-care bill was spent processing paper—$94 billion to process claims. It has been the author's experience that for any dental plan that is predominately traditional (fee-for-service oriented), claims processing costs and marketing expenses consume the greatest proportion of the administrative dollars (see Fig. 6–1).

The data systems of dental managed-care plans differ because they have no need to maintain expensive claims-based administrative data systems. Instead, less costly management information systems (MIS) are used that collect patient encounter data.

The difference is dramatic. Because traditional dental plans do not truly manage all aspects of dental care, the submission of claims and their subsequent processing is really the only way for the dental benefit plan to gather critical information. Dental claim forms are burdensome and time-consuming because there is a tremendous amount of administrative information required by the dental plan. Each claim form can be thought of as a combination of a beneficiary's statement and the dental provider's statement.

Weekly Average (98% of practices submit claims)		Weekly Median
Number of claims	59	48
Solo practice	44	—
Two dentists	70	—
Three or more dentists	130	—

Figure 6–1. Claim volume (Source: National Electronic Interchange Council, 1994)

BENEFICIARY'S STATEMENT ELEMENTS

- The patient is employed within the dental plan's service area
- If the person who received dental services is not the employee, then dependency must be established
- The employee received dental services thought to be covered services by the dental plan
- Providers are authorized by the employee to release information necessary to process the claim
- The dental plan is authorized to pay benefits to either the employee or directly to the dentist
- Identification of any other prospective third-party payers who would be liable for a portion of the claim and any current coordination-of-benefits provisions
- Authorization by the patient for review of claim by peer review organizations and/or dental-plan consultants
- Identify whether the patient is covered by Medicare
- Identify any condition covered by any governmental program, including details of the diagnosis and treatment for reimbursement and reporting requirements
- Adequate documentation accompanying the claim to establish the medical necessity of the dental services rendered

DENTAL PROVIDER'S STATEMENT ELEMENTS

- Indication of a federal tax identification number
- Verification that this provider rendered the services listed on the claim
- Provider is a licensed dentist at his or her practice location
- Provider rendered necessary dental services to the employee on a specific date for documented reasons

- Attestation that the employee is obligated to pay, and the dentist to collect, specific patient charges
- The dental condition treated is or is not job-related

Keep in mind that these elements are the minimum required—dental plans can and often do ask for more information, necessitating a myriad of claim forms and submission protocols that every practicing dentist has had to face.

WHAT IS ENCOUNTER DATA?

Every face-to-face diagnosis or treatment situation that a dentist has with a patient is termed an encounter. A record of exactly what happened during each patient encounter is called encounter data reporting.

Because the dental managed-care plan is so involved in managing the patient's total dental care, one would think that encounter data reporting would be more onerous than conventional claims processing. Just the opposite is true: since most primary care dentists are in a prospective payment arrangement (capitation), much of the financially oriented administrative data is already known to the dental plan. The author has seen encounter forms as simple as checklist-style "speedforms" with the provider's information preprinted on them. These forms are actually faster to complete than most handwritten drug prescriptions. Since the provider does not have to submit the forms as precedence for payment, the dental managed-care plan can collect them on a periodic basis. Separate documentation, such as radiographs, study models, and extensive treatment narratives, are not routinely necessary. A sample encounter data form might include:

- Date of service
- Patient's name
- Social security number
- Dependent number (if a dependent of the enrollee)
- Group number

- Preprinted ADA or HCPCS dental codes, by column, with quantity counts entered
- Co-payments collected
- Plan-specific codes and boxes to record broken appointments, no-shows, and late arrivals

Such forms often have room for 20 or more patients, making the old notion of one patient per claim form obsolete (see Fig. 6–2).

Some prepaid dental plans do not require encounter data reporting from their providers at all. In our definition of dental managed care, this position is not tenable. Encounter data reporting is easier and dramatically less obtrusive to the provider than conventional dental claim forms, and the data collected by plans are crucial. The main purpose behind encounter data collection is to capture dental service utilization data to support quality assurance evaluations and other reporting functions. Lack of this information causes the entire structure and process of managed care to collapse.

Utilization Review Systems

The collection of encounter data elements and subsequent processing by the dental managed-care plan's management information system yields many reports. One of the most critical to managed care involves those data elements that feed directly into a utilization review system (see Fig. 6–3).

Utilization review systems (also known as utilization management) help the dental plan to evaluate the medical necessity and appropriateness of dental services received by beneficiaries. These systems are designed to detect and report both underutilization and overutilization of dental services, use aggregate data to establish utilization patterns, conduct trend analysis, and develop statistical profiles of dental providers (also known as "practice profiling"). A typical utilization report compiled on a monthly basis might reflect the following information:

- Number of patients seen
- Number of patients enrolled

DENTAL PLAN

Patient Encounter Form

Provider Name: ____________

Provider Number: ____________

PATIENT NAME (LAST, FIRST)	DATE OF BIRTH MM–DD–YY	SOCIAL SECURITY # OR MEDI–CAL #	PATIENT SEX	TYPE OF VISIT CODE	TREATMENT DATE MM–DD–YY	ADA CODE	TOOTH NUMBER

TYPE OF VISIT CODES: (1) Initial (2) In Progress (3) Completion

Figure 6–2. Patient encounter form

```
                    ┌─────────────────┐
                    │ Member visits PCD│
                    └────────┬────────┘
                             │
                    ┌────────▼────────┐
                    │ PCD performs services│
                    │ and completes       │
                    │ encounter form      │
                    └────────┬────────┘
                             │
                    ┌────────▼────────┐
                    │ DMP enters information│
                    │ into MIS            │
                    └────────┬────────┘
          ┌──────────────────┼──────────────────┐
┌─────────▼────────┐ ┌───────▼────────┐ ┌───────▼────────┐
│ QA department    │ │ Provider relations│ │ UR personnel    │
│ receives data    │ │ discusses reports │ │ perform trend   │
│ for review       │ │ with providers    │ │ analysis        │
└──────────────────┘ └──────────────────┘ └──────────────────┘
```

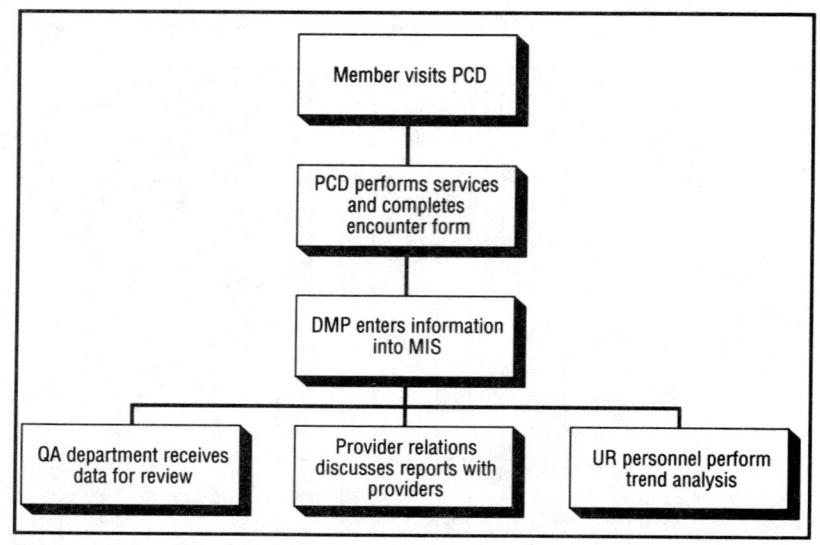

Figure 6–3. Sample utilization review system

- Utilization rate (overall)
- Total number of patient visits
- Number of new patients assigned
- Total number of reassignments (patients who ask to change providers)
- Total number of referrals
- Referral rate/100 patient visits
- Referral rate by specialty
- Referral rate of a PCD compared to his/her peers
- Frequency of specific procedures delivered
- Number of out-of-plan visits

Other areas of dental managed care can be readily evaluated, such as accessibility to services, appointment waiting times, and patient compliance. The resources consumed by an MIS designed for claims processing are enormous—the redirection of this power towards managing dental care holds great promise. The next step in this evolution is the elimination of paperwork entirely with the introduction of electronic claims submission (ECS) via electronic data interchange (EDI).

ELECTRONIC DATA INTERCHANGE AND ECS

The Netherlands has the greatest penetration of EDI in health-care systems of any other nation. In a country much smaller than ours, the Dutch Ministry of Health has estimated that EDI is saving from $10 million to $30 million per year in communication costs alone. EDI in the Netherlands includes electronic patient medical/dental records.

In the United States, dental plans are just now waking up to the benefits of paperless processing for both traditional and managed-care systems. The goal of all health-care EDI is the electronic transmission of all health-related transactions. Progressive dental offices can use their own computers to electronically "sweep" patient data for required encounter data elements, store the resulting electronic form, and transmit it over a telephone line to the dental plan. All of this takes but a fraction of the time and resources spent in filling out dental claim forms.

EDI depends on standardization to become truly cost-effective. The ANSI 837 standard defines a set of rules that binds together all of the required aspects of a health insurance claim. HCFA-1500 is a record format that performs a similar function for managed-care systems. Health-care EDI yields quality, speed, and cost reduction. Dental managed-care benefits from increased data accuracy, data that are more readily available for decision making, quality reviews, and strategic business planning. Fee-for-service plans will use EDI to simply automate their existing procedures—dental managed-care plans will reach for the stars.

When EDI advances to the point of facilitating real-time, health-care data interchange, every aspect of dentistry will benefit. EDI will eliminate delays from mailings and postal costs, provide immediate feedback on claims status, and facilitate instant payment of approved claims. Claims can be submitted as they are generated, thus eliminating delays due to batching cycles currently used by traditional dental plans.

The reduction in dental-plan personnel will dramatically lower administrative costs. Tremendous manpower is required in mailroom personnel, microfilm technicians, data-entry operators, claims auditors, dental-plan consultants, and fiduciary personnel. In theory, the resultant savings can be shared by all parties. Still, such a time is taking slow root in most American dental practices. As reported by Delta Dental Plan of Massachusetts, electronic claim submissions in 1993 were a paltry 10%. To catalyze dentists into bringing computers into their practices, Delta Dental Plan of Massachusetts is offering:

- Electronic Funds Transfer (EFT)
- Electronic explanation of benefits (on-line)
- Instant pretreatment estimates
- Ready capture of encounter data
- Instant verification of patient eligibility
- Daily feedback on patient balances

This stills leaves a problem for Delta and other dental-service organizations that have traditional dental plans—how does one deal with requirements for radiograph submission, study models, and the like? Radiographs can be electronically digitized, but only at great expense to the solo practitioner—equipment costs for this alone can dwarf the expense of an entire stand-alone personal computer.

As with other aspects of health-care reform, when one treatment delivery system benefits more from new technology than another, Darwinian principles start to work. Yes, EDI and electronic claims submission will result in cost savings for fee-for-service-based dental plans, but the real dividends will be realized by dental managed care.

CHAPTER 7

PROVIDER NETWORKS—IPAS AND THE LIKE

*"Faith! he must make his stories shorter
Or change his comrades once a quarter."*
JONATHAN SWIFT (1667–1745), ANGLO-IRISH SATIRIST. "VERSES ON THE DEATH OF DR. SWIFT," FROM *THE COLUMBIA DICTIONARY OF QUOTATIONS* (COLUMBIA UNIVERSITY PRESS, 1993).

Dental managed-care plans will make or break their reputations in the marketplace at the hands of their provider networks. Knowing the laws and demands of the free market, the integrity, quality, and professionalism of a plan's provider network will either be a badge of honor or an embarrassment not readily overcome.

Maxwell Davis and Benjamin Schechter had this to say:

> *The HMO concept is designed to promote change and brings together two classic American virtues: private initiative and monetary incentive. No person is forced to*

form an HMO and no provider is forced to work for an HMO. An HMO can be sponsored by a variety of agencies. Dentists can be paid on a fee-for-service basis, on a salary basis, or on a capitation basis. They could work under one roof as in the group practice (staff model) or alone in their own offices, such as in the primary care network or as an independent practice association (IPA). Many, if not most dentists who establish solo practices are not likely to participate in HMOs of the staff-model type. That is why the development of the IPA offers the greatest opportunity for the solo-practicing dentist to provide care through the HMO mechanism.[20]

All of us need to keep in mind that while the term "dental HMO" makes for a very nice moniker, in reality no dental plan can ever become a federally qualified (or recognized) health maintenance organization. When Dr. Paul Elwood first coined the term during the Nixon administration, the resulting HMO Act of 1973 was intended only for those plans intending to offer a full scope of health-care services. Dental-only plans are considered specialized plans, and as such cannot be included in the act. The term "dental maintenance organization" (DMO) is growing in popularity and is proper in this context.

Nonetheless, in many medical circles the terms "managed care" and "HMO" are synonymous. This can lead to confusion when medical HMO terms are used to describe provider networks. Reviewing the legal descriptions as put forth by the federal Health Care Financing Administration will clarify things greatly.

STAFF MODEL

"This is an arrangement in which you employ health professionals to provide health services to members. These professionals:

- Are subject to your staff policies,
- Engage in the coordinated practice of their professions,
- Furnish health services you have contracted to provide to members,

- Share medical records, equipment, and professional, technical, and administrative staff, and

- Provide their professional services in accordance with a compensation arrangement, other than fee-for-service, which you establish."[21]

GROUP PRACTICE

"This is a partnership, association, corporation, or other legal structure that is composed of health professionals licensed to practice medicine. Other licensed health professionals, such as dentists, may participate in the group. Group members include health professionals who are engaged as partners, associates, or shareholders in the group practice. A majority of the members of the group practice must be physicians. Members of the group are also expected to:

- Pool their income and distribute it according to a prearranged salary or other plan unrelated to the provision of specific health services;

- Share medical records, major equipment, and professional, technical, and administrative staff;

- Have substantial responsibility (over 35% of their collective professional activity) for the delivery of health services to your members; and

- Establish an arrangement whereby a member's enrollment status is not known to the health professional who provides health services to the member (i.e., welfare, private-pay, etc.)"[22]

INDIVIDUAL PRACTICE ASSOCIATION (IPA)

"This is a partnership, association, corporation, or other legal entity that delivers or arranges for the delivery of health services. The IPA has written services arrangements or contracts with health professionals. These written services provide:

- A description of the services that these health professionals provide
- The compensation arrangements
- Procedures for sharing, to the extent feasible, health and other records, equipment, and professional, technical, and administrative staff."[23]

While the expense, financial requirements, and administrative workload of running a full-blown dental benefit plan may appear daunting, forming an IPA is, in essence, a bite-sized version that dentists may find valuable as managed-care systems increase in popularity.

As with all delivery care systems associated with managed care, there are common characteristics:

- Providers are under contract to provide care for a specific group of patients
- Contracts provide for a specific reimbursement mechanism, often modified by provider type (PCD or specialist)
- Contracts impose certain limits and exclusions on the patient's care
- Contracts provide for termination from participation
- Quality reviews and utilization reviews are mandated
- Providers are free to participate in other programs
- Providers enter into at-risk contracts

Additionally, dentists who successfully form an IPA will go through a sequence of events not unlike dental benefit-plan development. These events involve:

1. Completing surveys of purchasers, potential patients, and providers
2. Establishing operating parameters (e.g., scope of benefits, deductibles, co-payments, and benefit maximums)

3. Formalizing plan development; legal descriptions and licensing requirements

4. Developing reimbursement mechanisms to panel providers

5. Building a provider panel

6. Finding a suitable administrator to handle claims processing and reviews

7. Finding a carrier willing to market the IPA

Independent practice associations allow health-care providers a means of controlling situations that historically were entirely handled by dental service plans. The American Dental Association offers excellent information and limited support for those dentists interested in this area. Another fine source of information can be found by networking with medical colleagues involved in their own IPA networks.

Rather than directly marketing their IPA, many dentists prefer to establish an IPA in partnership with a dental managed-care plan that desires a provider network in their area. This strategy is discussed in detail later in this chapter.

MIXED MODELS

As the title suggests, mixed-model networks are those in which both staff-model and IPA-model situations coexist. A common occurrence is when dental-plan-operated clinics already exist, but new provider networks are needed in areas of service-area expansions. When the areas are geographically isolated, there is little problem with mixed-model forms of DMOs.

Where staff-model facilities and the private offices of network providers coexist in close proximity, there is always the opportunity for conflict of interest to occur, in which the dental managed-care plan preferentially assigns patients to plan-owned-and-operated facilities. Contracts between the DMO and network providers should spell out patient assignment procedures in absolute clarity to avoid even the semblance of favoritism.

DIRECT SERVICE CONTRACTS

"These are contracts between you and a health provider who is not a member of your staff or an entity that is not a medical group or IPA for the provision of health services to your members. These contracts are similar to service agreements with medical IPAs."[24]

Most dentists will enter into direct provider contracts with dental managed-care plans. Note that for our medical colleagues, the majority has elected to band together in other forms of practice arrangements. A discussion of the dental IPA as an effective practice arrangement comes later in this chapter.

For the time being, we need to discuss that the entryway into a provider network (whatever form it acquires) requires several steps:

1. Completion of a formal application to join the network

2. Completion of a dental facility checklist (see Table 7–1)

3. Completion of an on-site office audit by dental plan personnel

Many dentists find this entire process strange and confusing, and some are even hostile to the idea of an audit. Keep in mind that the dental managed-care plan is obligated to ensure the professionalism of its provider network—these steps are actually the providers' introduction to the plan's quality assurance program. Since each quality assurance program must assess elements dealing with structure, process, and outcome, the auditing of a provider's office entails both structure (the facility itself) and process (chart review and patient screenings).

APPLICATION PROCESS

Dental managed-care plans need to have knowledge of your practice and all providers at an office site who wish to participate. A typical application form might have the following categories of information:

- General information—name(s), address(es), phone number(s)
- Type of practice—solo or group, PCD or specialist

Table 7–1
Preenrollment Dental Facility Checklist.

YES	NO	N/A	EVALUATION CRITERIA	COMMENTS
			I. **ADMINISTRATION** 1. Process for emergencies—triage protocol. 2. Protocol for follow-up of broken appointments. 3. Protocol for specialty referrals. 4. Plan office procedure manual on-site. 5. Procedure for reviewing patients' complaints or grievances on-site and by plan is in place. 6. Scheduled appointments available. 7. Waiting time to see provider is reasonable. 8. Personnel have Hep. B immunizations or being offered at expense of provider. Documentation required. 9. Exam by dentist and X-rays prescribed prior to taking of initial X-rays. II. **ACCESSIBILITY** 1. Parking is adequate. 2. Handicapped parking is available. 3. Office Hours: M _____ T _____ W _____ T _____ F _____ SA _____ SU _____ Lunch: _____ 4. Provisions made for evening and after-hour communication and services. 5. Restroom facilities and building accessible to the handicapped. III. **FACILITY AND EQUIPMENT** 1. Space in facility is adequate. 2. Facility and equipment clean, safe, neat, and well maintained. 3. Amalgamators covered—prevent spillage of mercury. 4. Spill kit available if bulk mercury is used. 5. Scrap amalgam stored under appropriate liquid in a tightly closed container.	

YES	NO	N/A	EVALUATION CRITERIA	COMMENTS
			6. Prescription drugs stored in a place inaccessible to patients and logged if dispensed on-site. 7. Needles, syringes, prescription pads stored securely. 8. OSHA Manual and other OSHA requirements met (posters). **IV. EMERGENCY PROCEDURES AND EQUIPMENT** 1. Dental emergency kit available, appropriately stocked, no expired items, labeled with an inventory of medications. 2. First-aid kit available. 3. Staff aware of location of emergency kits, their contents, and general use of medications. 4. Portable emergency oxygen available, tank full, with positive pressure valve and ambu bag, personnel trained in use. 5. Facility has a written emergency action plan in response to fire and other disasters. Staff is knowledgeable regarding procedures to be followed. 6. Directions to exits are marked, if the exit is not readily apparent. Doors are marked NO EXIT if not an egress and possibility of confusion exists. 7. Easily accessible eye-wash stations installed and operative, and personnel trained in their use. **V. RADIOLOGY** 1. Type(s) of X-ray machine: [ ] Intra-oral; [ ] Panographic. 2. X-ray units registered. Certificate available. 3. Lead apron intact (with thyroid collar) for patients. 4. Required radiology poster displayed.	

YES	NO	N/A	EVALUATION CRITERIA	COMMENTS
			VI. LICENSES AND CERTIFICATES 1. Names of all dentists working at the facility posted. 2. Licenses and certificates for all dentists, hygienists, and support staff available and current. PROFESSIONALS: Dentist and Hygienist License; RDA Licenses for auxiliaries; X-ray for X-ray techs, etc. OTHER: DEA, expanded duties, RDH. **VII. STERILIZATION AND INFECTION CONTROL** 1. Type of sterilization procedures used: [ ] Autoclave; [ ] Chemi-clave; [ ] Dry heat; [ ] Chemical sterilants, name(s) _____ 2. Staff is knowledgeable in sterilization procedures, heat vs. cold sterilization; sterilization vs. disinfecting. 3. Protocols posted for sterilization procedures. 4. Staff wears gloves, masks, protective attire and eyewear appropriately. 5. Instruments for invasive procedures (i.e., surgery curettages, etc.) bagged dated, heat sterilized, and remain bagged until used. 6. Chemical indicators are on outside of all sterilized packs and have changed colors appropriately to verify process. 7. Packs torn/damaged, wet, expiration date exceeded, or when sterility is questioned, are not used. 8. Heat sterilizers spore tested at least weekly and results kept as a log. 9. Cold sterilization containers labeled with name, dilution, and expiration date of solution. 10. Sharps—deposited in a rigid container, leak and puncture proof, tightly lidded to preclude loss of contents.	

YES	NO	N/A	EVALUATION CRITERIA	COMMENTS
			11. Infectious waste and contaminated waste placed in appropriate receptacles with biohazard signs and disposed of appropriately.	
			12. Infection control procedures followed in the office laboratory (i.e., pumice pan, disinfection of impressions, dentures and other appliances going to or coming from the outside laboratory).	
			13. Contaminated instruments properly cleaned prior to sterilization. Utility gloves used. Ultrasonic recommended.	
			14. Disinfection of hard surfaces in operatory between patients, and at end of day with EPA-approved solution.	
			15. Handpieces and curettage tips are heat sterilized after each use.	
			16. Handpieces and water lines are flushed appropriately.	
			17. Anti-retraction valves have been installed to dental-unit water lines.	
			18. Contaminated laundry is handled and laundered appropriately.	

- Hours of operation

- Services offered

- Emergency coverage—including details on after-hour coverage

- Office staff—number, types, and full-time or part-time status

- Office information—queries about the functioning of your office, allowing the plan's network specialist(s) to determine patient capacity and current workload

- Treatment facilities—numbers of operatories, lab space, etc.

- Regulatory compliance—usually a checklist of OSHA requirements

- Payment provisions—the plan's assessment of your current mixture of patients and plans, special credit arrangements, etc.
- Provider information—details on education, licensure status, DEA number, hospital affiliations, and professional memberships
- Copy of declarations page from current professional liability carrier

After routine processing of a provider's application (with time for appropriate inquiries of the state licensing board, and perhaps the National Practitioner Data Bank), the provider will be notified of a need to schedule the actual office visit by plan personnel.

Typically, an audit team from the dental managed-care plan will schedule a specific day and time to perform the audit. It does not have to be a surprise inspection—remember that by this time, your application has been accepted, but the audit team must assure itself that your office facility meets minimum standards (as shown on the checklist) prior to final approval. The team will usually consist of a dental auxiliary trained in office audits and environmental health and safety/infection control techniques and will conduct the majority of the facility (structure) inspection. A dental consultant will generally round out the team and will be concentrating on a random review of your dental records (process) (see Table 7–2).

Table 7–2
Dental Record Assessment Form.

PLAN _____   DATE _____
FACILITY _____   AUDITOR _____
PATIENT RECORDS REVIEWED:

AUDIT NUMBER	PATIENT NAME	CHART NUMBER	RATING
1			
2			
3			
4			
5			
6			
7			
8			
9			
10			

CATEGORY	SCORE	TOTAL	RATING
PT. NO	1 2 3 4 5 6 7 8 9 10		S/U

1. CONSENT FORM
    a. Informed consent
    b. Signed and dated
2. MEDICAL/DENTAL HISTORY
    a. Adequate data base
    b. Information complete
    c. Medical alert
    d. Evaluated, initialed, dated by D.D.S.
    e. Patient signature
    f. Update on recall
    g. Chief complaint recorded
3. EXTRA/INTRA ORAL EXAM
    a. Existing conditions/restorations/appliances recorded symbolically
    b. Status of teeth
    c. Status of soft tissue
4. RADIOGRAPHS
    a. Quality
    b. Quantity
    c. Document critical structures
    d. Initial X-rays prescribed by D.D.S.
    e. Frequency
    f. Current, dated
5. DIAGNOSIS
    a. Caries
    b. Periodontic
    c. Endodontic
    d. Consistent with complaint, history, and objective findings
6. TREATMENT PLAN
    a. Proposed treatment plan recorded
    b. Recall treatment plan, if necessary
    c. Sequenced
    d. Appropriate

CATEGORY	SCORE	TOTAL	RATING
PT. NO	1 2 3 4 5 6 7 8 9 10		S/U

7. PREVENTIVE SERVICES
   a. Prophys scheduled appropriately
   b. Oral hygiene instructions recorded
   c. Fluoride treatments and sealants provided as necessary

8. TREATMENT QUALITY
   a. Operative
   b. Prosthetics
   c. Endodontics
   d. Periodontics
   e. Emergency treatment
   f. Other

9. PROGRESS NOTES
   a. Chronological/N.V. notations
   b. All treatment services identified
   c. Prescriptions completely documented, including Sig.
   d. Legible
   e. Anesthetics documented
   f. Tooth numbers, surfaces, and type of restoration recorded
   g. Medications and materials identified

10. TREATMENT
    a. Appropriate sequence
    b. Medical consultations when necessary
    c. Specialty referrals appropriate
    d. Timely, efficient

11. CONTINUITY OF CARE
    a. Canceled/failed appointments, follow-up documented
    b. Specialist referrals noted

CATEGORY	SCORE	TOTAL	RTING
PT. NO	1 2 3 4 5 6 7 8 9 10		S/U
c. Follow-up of referrals			
d. Recalls documented			
12. MANAGEMENT OF PATIENT			
a. Outcome			
b. Overall patient care			

RATING

COMMENTS

SCORING			RATING BY COMPONENT
S SATISFACTORY		+1	S = +1 to +10
N NEUTRAL OR NOT APPLICABLE		N/A	TEN RECORDS {
U UNSATISFACTORY		− 1	U = 0 to − 10

RATING BY CATEGORY

SATISFACTORY

Indicates clinical quality and/or facilities and/or professional performance rated in the range of excellence. No deficiencies found.

Indicates clinical quality and/or facilities and/or professional performance rated in the range of acceptance. Deficiencies identified were not a pattern and did not affect the well-being of patients.

UNSATISFACTORY

Indicates clinical quality and/or facilities and/or professional performance which should be repeated, replaced, repaired, or corrected for preventive reasons and is likely to cause future damage to the patient's general or dental health or to individual components of the patient's masticatory system.

Indicates clinical quality and/or professional performance that MUST be repeated, replaced, and/or immediately treated because damage is now occurring or because serious inadequacies exist.

The checklists shown are examples of two in current use—dental plans may have many variations of them. The checklists should be made available to the dental provider well in advance of the office audit. This will allow the provider and his or her staff to familiarize themselves with those audit criteria that the plan's audit team will use, and perhaps perform some early corrections. The point of the audits is to ensure quality, adequate office space for future assigned patients, handicap access, etc., and make any corrections needed prior to assigning patients to the office.

The dental consultant will be reviewing the dental records for many things, including (but not limited to):

- Organization
- Legibility
- Dated entries (including procedures performed)
- Signed entries
- Treating provider identified on each procedure
- Diagnosis
- Treatment plan
- Drugs prescribed
- Allergies (with separate notation on external surface of chart)
- Medication list (if applicable)
- Emergency information
- Informed consent
- Dental history and updates
- Medical history and updates
- Case management and referral information filed in a timely manner
- Notation of any cultural/linguistic needs
- Charting of any examination findings requiring follow-up and recalls

While at a provider's office, audit teams are expected to collect data, not to perform the final analysis and corrections (if needed). Final tabulations, discussions, and analysis will be performed back at the plan's business office. The audit team may be running on a tight schedule, especially in areas where the dental managed-care plan is expanding into new service areas and having to audit many new provider offices. Accordingly, the prospective network provider should not press for a final decision on the spot, for no audit team can properly render one.

The findings of the audit team will, in most plans, be routed past the eyes of the dental director and QA committee. A final report will then be prepared. Within a matter of days to weeks (depending on the size of the provider network), the dentist should receive notification of the final audit results, recommendations, and decisions (see Fig. 7–1).

More times than not, the audit will reveal that the provider's office is in substantial compliance, and nothing further will need to be done. If the audit team discovers one or more areas of serious deficiencies, then a corrective action plan (CAP) will be created. This CAP is intended to alert the dentist as to:

1. what violations were present at the day of the audit, as well as
2. what specific actions will be required to bring the facility into full compliance.

Only in the most severe cases of noncompliance (or an office's failure of a second audit) would the provider face possible refusal of inclusion into the provider network.

INDEPENDENT PRACTICE ASSOCIATIONS AND PROVIDER NETWORKS

Despite the growing numbers of dentists electing to join a dental managed-care plan's provider network, many prefer to hold back some autonomy and increase their bargaining power. This is especially valuable in those areas of the nation where several managed-care plans are

Dear Dr. Quattlebaum:

The results of your recent office audit have reached my desk, and I am pleased to announce that, once again, you are in "substantial compliance." Additionally, our DMO consultant, Dr. Detail, was very impressed with the results of your recent office expansion. DMO is looking forward to assigning more patients to you.

Dr. Detail has noted that the absence of medical alerts on some charts might be due to the chart conversion that is currently underway. She did note that the initial charting that shows the condition of the mouth at the initial visit was missing; a sample copy of your new charts showed a provision for this information, and it should be included for your DMO patients.

I am sending you a copy of an informed consent form used at other DMO offices for endodontic treatment. Courts have ruled that nonroutine dental care, such as endodontia, periodontia, and oral surgery are not considered routine. Please call Provider Relations for some or all of these forms—DMO is pleased to supply them to you.

Concerning Mr. Next, Dr. Detail noted that #19 was missing, but the replacement for this tooth was not addressed in the treatment plan. Also, on Ms. Winters, #14 had gross decay distally under a crown, and #30 was missing with replacement not addressed. Remember that DMO allows the replacement of a space with either fixed or removable prostheses based on your judgment and the patient's wishes. If none of the above patients desires tooth replacement at this time, please note this in the master dental record.

I hope to see the office before your next review in March. If not, I hope to see you next week at our special seminar series for network providers.

Sincerely,

M.C. Progressive, D.D.S.
Dental Director
DMO

Figure 7–1. Sample audit results review letter

vying for the available dentists within a certain geographic service area, especially rural areas where managed care has special difficulties.

The American Dental Association defines an independent practice association (also called "individual practice association") as "a legal entity organized and governed by individual participating dentists for the primary purpose of collectively entering into contracts to provide dental services to enrolled populations."

In the structure of an IPA, dentists may see any patient—IPA-related or not. Thus, IPAs are less restrictive to the dentist than closed panel arrangements and similar variations.

The exciting part about joining or helping to build an independent practice association is that benefit designs, claims administration, and patient/provider relations programs are developed and administered by the practicing dentists themselves.

All of this is not without a price. Dentists who are part of an IPA must provide the initial outlay of capital needed for operational expenses and must share the insurance risk as the IPA manages contracts.

For many dentists who actively participate in an IPA, there is simply no better option. Since the dentists are legally and financially at-risk, an IPA is considered a safe harbor from most antitrust law scenarios. In the infamous case of *Arizona v. Maricopa County Medical Society,* a group of providers found themselves in serious violation of federal law simply by agreeing on a minimum fee schedule amongst themselves. Independent practice associations allow for free discussions of fees, benefit levels, and related issues as they pertain to the business of the IPA.

Dealing with an established IPA can be a distinct advantage for the purchaser of dental benefits. A well-managed IPA offers:

- Professional management

- Practicing dentists with financial stake in success of the association

- "Turnkey" network with greater acceptance by other dentists

An IPA established in a service area prior to the emergence of a dental managed-care plan can be an attractive situation for both parties. The dental managed-care plan sees a ready-made provider network in place, avoiding most of the high costs involved in establishing new provider networks. The IPA that boasts professional management can position itself to negotiate better contracts and agreements for its member-dentists.

If the dentist is considering participation in an existing IPA, keep these questions in mind:

- Does this IPA truly have professional management (i.e., a third-party administrator)?
- Are there indications of a "sham" IPA, where dentists are restricted from participating in other programs?
- Is the IPA membership so large that its market share threatens legal action from other dental plans (generally a concern when more than 35% of the area's providers are involved in the IPA)?
- Does the state's department of insurance (or other appropriate state regulatory agency) have any adverse actions pending against the IPA?

Within the dental benefits arena, independent practice associations offer the dentist an opportunity to take a proactive, enriching approach to the world of managed care. For the dentist who is not adverse to accepting a reasonable amount of risk, and is confident in his or her practice decisions, then consideration of an IPA is a must.

THE LEGAL WAR OVER "ANY WILLING PROVIDER"

As Dr. Shuwarger related in a previous chapter, there are times when a provider, content with a traditional-style practice, is forced to seek participation in managed care. Yet, he may find himself in a situation where there is "no room on the boat." As more and more providers of all professions face this reality, legal challenges have sprung up to end any restrictive practices.

From a purely business standpoint, dental managed-care plans in many (mostly metropolitan) areas do not want every possible dental provider as part of their network. When a dental plan selects certain providers and excludes others, it creates a form of managed competition in the marketplace.

By contracting with every provider, the dental plan would soon lose any cost benefit. Bargaining power between plan and providers, competing for limited places in a particular network, is also lost. In essence, being forced to contract with every licensed provider is no different from a traditional indemnity plan.

The March 28, 1994 issue of *Medicine & Health* reported that 18 states are considering some form of "any willing provider" law. Managed-care plans and others who deal with provider networks would be prevented from excluding any provider that was willing to accept the same provider agreement terms and conditions as was offered to the current network providers. A proposal that was making the rounds in the Florida legislature would force plans to hire any willing provider that accepts *less* than the plan's usual reimbursement rate.

Managed-care groups claim that these laws violate a main tenet of managed-care arrangements—the negotiation of favorable payment arrangements with a limited number of providers in exchange for an assured patient volume. In 1994, the National Governor's Conference released a position paper against the establishment of "any willing provider" laws, claiming that they would derail any health-care reform movement at a state level.

Accordingly, most health-care reform packages discussed earlier do not allow for "any willing provider" laws. They would preempt any such laws at the federal level in the quest for managed competition between health-care plans and the preservation of a free market.

The dentist considering the managed-care marketplace needs to understand that although a well-run dental managed-care plan can offer substantial benefits to providers chosen for its network, there may not be room for all providers in a particular service area. Providers must not waste time in assessing a dental managed-care plan's offer to join a provider network. Adopting a wait-and-see attitude can result in a lost opportunity to participate, with the possible resultant loss of many patients.

CHAPTER 8

SPECIAL CONCERNS FOR THE DENTAL SPECIALIST

*"No atomic physicist has to worry,
people will always want to kill other people on a mass scale.
Sure, he's got the fridge full of sausages and spring water."*
WILLIAM BURROUGHS (1914–), U.S. AUTHOR.
"A WORD TO THE WISE GUY," *THE ADDING MACHINE: COLLECTED ESSAYS* (1985) FROM *THE COLUMBIA DICTIONARY OF QUOTATIONS* (COLUMBIA UNIVERSITY PRESS, 1993).

In a recent article appearing in the *Sacramento Business Journal,* one orthopedic surgeon was lamenting about the role of specialists in a managed-care provider network. The problem, in his mind, was not that a certain managed-care plan would never get every orthopedic surgeon in Sacramento to contract with their network, but rather that the managed-care plan could only use three or four of them in their network anyway. Indeed, several of his colleagues had left the area due to a drying-up of available patients.

As a board-certified periodontist, I know that dental specialists have to wrestle with two things. The first is pleasing the referring general dentist—the second is pleasing the patients themselves. In more recent times, specialists have had to be increasingly sensitive to economic constraints imposed by the patient's particular dental benefit program. In periodontics, it is quite easy to reach the usual benefit maximum in a fee-for-service plan during the initial course of therapy. Doing so can leave the patient with little or no financial resources to complete other therapies with the general dentist.

With the advent of PPOs, dental plans simply had to duplicate their provider panels—one for primary care and another for specialty care. Discounted fees were negotiated on both sides, and the general dentists in the PPO were limited in their referrals to the specialists in the specialty panel.

Managed care will dramatically alter even this arrangement. The dental specialist will increasingly discover that his long-nurtured relationships with referring dentists can only persist if both specialist and PCD are under contract to the same managed-care plan. Even at that, there is no guarantee that the PCD will be able to direct his or her referrals to any one particular specialist.

In order to adequately monitor the utilization of services and appropriateness of specialty care, the PCD may not be able to refer directly to another plan specialist. More often than not, the PCD will have to initiate a referral request, and that request will require approval by the managed-care dental plan.

To the chagrin of most dental specialists, many prepaid dental plans force their PCDs through some incredible ordeals to accomplish a referral. Consider these examples:

- Endodontics—one plan expects only molars to require referral. The referral request mandates that individual radiographs, full-mouth radiographs, and study models be sent to the dental director for authorization.

- Periodontics—another plan requires two full-mouth scaling and root planings be performed six months apart by the PCD; if periodontitis persists three to six months after the second round of S/RPs were rendered, the referral can be initiated.

- Children under age three—still another plan requires the PCD to attempt treatment on *three different occasions* before initiating a referral; and flatly states that any child patient older than three years of age who remains a behavioral problem may be taken to a pediatric dentist *at the PCD's personal expense!*

On a brighter note, reimbursement of the specialist is usually more accommodating than for the PCD, for whom capitation is the predominant form of reimbursement. According to Evelyn Ireland, Executive Director of the National Association of Prepaid Dental Plans (NAPDP), one member plan has as many as 12 different compensation systems for its providers.[25] Various compensation methods for specialists include fixed co-payment, discounted UCR, and co-payment and UCR, among others (see Fig. 8–1).

Dental specialists tend to make common mistakes when faced with the growth of managed care. One may stop cultivating new referral sources; another may consider relocating. If you are a dental specialist

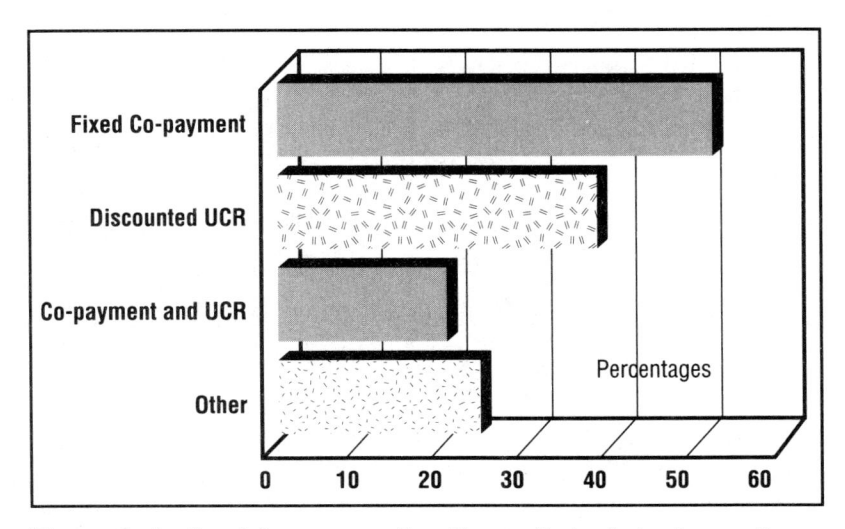

Figure 8–1. Specialty compensation (Source:Evelyn Ireland, executive director of the National Association of Prepaid Dental Plans, personal correspondence, 9 June 1994)

who is willing to face the future of managed care, there are definite strategies that can place you in a very favorable position should "managed care come to town."

POINT 1:
CONTINUE TO ACTIVELY MARKET YOUR SERVICES AND EXPAND YOUR REFERRAL BASE

Not only is this good strategy in the fee-for-service environment, but it also makes perfect sense in managed care. Dental managed-care plans will be known by the quality and completeness of their provider networks. Plans may approach general dentists and pediatric dentists at first, when service areas are being defined and the primary care network is being formed. These new PCDs may have critical input to the dental plan in regard to what specialists should be offered contracts or agreements. You will want your name to be as prominent then as it is now.

POINT 2:
ASSURE YOUR CURRENT REFERRING DENTISTS THAT YOU ARE WILLING TO CONSIDER FOLLOWING THEM INTO A MANAGED-CARE NETWORK

In this strategy, you treat the referring dentist as a partner. And in business, partners review all new ventures together. You may decide to split the legal costs of having contracts reviewed or the cost of bringing in an outside consultant. The dental plan can benefit by having a turnkey referral team, and the contractual terms might be sweeter as a result.

POINT 3:
CONTACT THOSE MANAGED CARE PLANS ALREADY OPERATING IN YOUR AREA

Begin a dialogue with a provider network specialist from each dental managed-care plan regardless of whether their network currently needs another specialist or not. Letting plans know that you are interested in possible participation doesn't obligate the specialist to anything—but it will allow you time to study the various managed-care plans, placing yourself in a better negotiating position in the future.

POINT 4:
CONSIDER FORMING A MULTISPECIALTY PRACTICE WITH OTHER SPECIALISTS

In many areas of the country, dental specialists are forming multispecialty practices in record numbers. First, there is a definite economy of scale that will always benefit a group practice over a solo practice. Second, dental plans are naturally drawn to those group practices that can offer one-stop shopping for specialty care. The key here is to be a multispecialty practice. It is fine to add additional oral surgeons, endodontists, etc., in time as the practice grows, but the initial appeal (and value) is to cover all of the dental specialties with appropriate numbers of providers.

POINT 5:
CONSIDER SUBSPECIALIZING

Unlike the medical profession, dentistry does not formally recognize subspecialties. However, there are legions of dentists who restrict their practice to hospital dentistry, treatment of special-needs patients, home-based care patients, and so on. In business, they would be known as niche providers, for they provide a service that the rank-and-file providers are not equipped (or not willing) to handle. For those dental managed-care plans with broad scope of benefits, subspecialists can be a powerful addition to a provider network.

POINT 6:
PUSH YOUR SPECIALTY ORGANIZATION INTO TAKING AN ACTIVE ROLE IN DENTAL MANAGED CARE

Just as the specialists themselves must adapt to the changing dental practice environment, so should their respective specialty academies and certifying boards. These organizations must be vigilant in both the numbers of specialists trained and the breadth of their training. Dentistry, unlike medicine, does not benefit from ever-increasing numbers of specialists. Additionally, dental specialty organizations will need to closely examine their role within a provider network and orient their institutional marketing programs accordingly. These same associations can issue statements condemning the types of restrictions on specialty referrals mentioned previously.

Remember that in dentistry, specialists remain in the minority of dental providers. This is to our profession's benefit, as the generalist-to-specialist ratio is closer to what medical managed care is attempting to achieve. Since we are closer to the ideal balance, we owe it to ourselves and our profession to maintain this strength.

Chapter 9

Making Room for Managed Care in Your Practice

"They are ill discoverers that think there is no land when they see nothing but sea."
Francis Bacon (1561–1626), English philosopher, essayist, statesman. *The Advancement of Learning*, Bk. 2, ch. 7, sct. 5 (1605) from *The Columbia Dictionary of Quotations* (Columbia University Press, 1993).

Dental managed care will never really work for providers, purchasers, or patients unless all parties are satisfied with the process. Some dentists are steadfastly opposed to anything resembling managed care and refuse to participate. Others see dental managed care as a practice reality (like it or not) and worry about whether they and their practice can adapt to it.

This chapter is written for those dentists who fear that their participation in dental managed care is akin to being a "square peg in a round hole." Nothing could be further from the truth. In the practice of law, the process of discovery often produces the truth. Providers who discover similarities between their own philosophy of dentistry and that of managed care will also find truth.

Take another look at the three basic elements of managed care:

- Access to dental care
- Delivery of quality dental care
- Cost-effectiveness of dental treatment

Let's review them singly and within the perspective of a dental practice.

ACCESS TO DENTAL CARE

What dentist does not want patients to have access to his or her professional services? We carefully consider which communities have a need for our services when deciding to establish a dental practice. Office space is secured, with attention given to prominence, adequate parking, access for the handicapped, and similar concerns.

We join dental societies and begin to network with our colleagues. Marketing decisions are made, advertising methods are decided upon, and staff are trained—not to scare patients away, but to attract them to a new and growing practice.

Managed care has a similar goal. Dentists often consider managed care as promoting limited access. In reality, it is just the opposite. Consider a patient who has obtained dental benefits through his or her employer. The dental plan administering the benefit program may or may not be financially attractive to dentists located close to the patient. In this situation, the patient may encounter problems in finding a dentist willing to treat him or her given that the patient wants to use their dental benefits program to the greatest extent possible.

Dental plans that allow for any licensed dentist to become a participating provider do not guarantee that every dentist will elect to participate. The dental plan can help steer a patient towards participating providers in his or her area, but nothing ensures that a dentist will be found that can see that patient on a regular basis.

For this patient, freedom of choice technically exists, but access to a dentist remains elusive. This patient may have only emergency needs met, obtain sporadic, episodic care, and never receive true case management. The traditional dental plan can only provide a payment mechanism after a dentist is found and after treatment is received.

Dental managed care seeks out those providers who demonstrate good dental-practice management skills. These providers are able to commit themselves to caring for a number of assigned patients, as well as accommodate other classifications of patients. Patients who are enrolled in a dental managed-care plan no longer have to find a dentist—they are able to choose one from within a provider network, or be assigned to one by the managed care plan. What is mistaken for limited access is in reality guaranteed access by virtue of prenegotiations with an adequate number of providers.

DELIVERY OF QUALITY DENTAL CARE

Patients judge the quality of the dental care that they receive differently than do the dentists themselves. Patients tend to judge the dental treatment experience in subjective terms (painless visits, courteous staff, gentle dentists) while dentists are taught to focus on the technical skills (marginal integrity of restorations, accuracy of impressions, etc.). There is not a single practicing dentist who has not faced a difficult patient who did not appreciate the treatment experience despite technically superior results. Providers find themselves indulging in dental clichés such as "good patients breed good dentistry," or the nearly morbid "patients are the enemy." Difficult patients often complain to the dental plan, their employer, and their friends, which can become a practice liability.

Dental managed care avoids many of the patient's uncertainties by providing a practice environment in which patients are assured that the dentists who belong to a provider network have:

- Passed a preenrollment on-site audit
- Been carefully credentialed by the dental managed-care plan

- Been required to participate in quality assurance activities

Dentists in current, active practices maintain their licensure by taking continuing education courses. Most would seek to improve their professional skills despite such requirements. Offices are adorned with certificates, plaques, and diplomas, all attesting to the provider's skill and qualifications.

The pursuit of excellence is as much a part of dentistry as any other notable profession. What dentists usually fear is that monitoring, audits, and visits by managed-care plans will become punitive.

The best of the dental managed-care plans will be proud of their provider networks and will seek preservation over exploitation. If these plans abused their own provider network, what would regulatory agencies do to them in return? What actions would a purchaser take if he or she had evidence that quality of care was being ignored? Reestablishing provider networks is an expensive proposition for any dental managed-care plan—it makes greater business sense to keep a good one humming along.

Dental managed care establishes linkages between providers for the purposes of education, correction of problems, and reinforcement of positive outcomes that preserves the integrity of the provider network. Dental plans exist by selling a product. To a well-managed dental plan, the provider network is the key to selling that product. Whatever degrades the product degrades the commercial viability of the dental managed-care plan. Accordingly, the smart dental managed-care plans nurture their provider networks.

COST-EFFECTIVENESS OF DENTAL TREATMENT

Gold is better than silver. Silicone impression material is more accurate than alginate. The skill level of the dentist remains constant whether the treatment consists of amalgam restorations or precious-metal cast restorations, or the impression is made with alginate or a silicone-based product. The dentist uses his or her skills to provide the best treatment result, or outcome, that is achievable given the limitations of the materials or products used.

In the unique marketplace of dental patients, not everyone can afford gold. Not every patient desires gold, as many patients allow cosmetic demands to override concerns over restoration longevity, marginal adaptation, and periodontal health. Patients and purchasers, when faced with financial pressures, often want what is appropriate rather than ideal. Dentistry, unlike medicine, has a high degree of discretionary treatment options available for the patient. These options can all yield positive treatment outcomes without being labeled as inferior treatment by the dentist.

Dental managed care strives to conserve resources by providing a quality service at a price that the marketplace will accept. Providers are under no obligation to provide the most expensive services simply because the assigned patients are not charged fees, any more than a dentist must provide them under traditional plans. The principle of LEPEAT[26] comes into play—provide the patient with the **least expensive, professionally ethical, alternative treatment.** If a given array of alternative treatments will result in a healthier patient, then the LEPEAT principle will not be in conflict with established professional ethics.

GUIDELINES FOR MAKING DENTAL PRACTICES COST-EFFECTIVE

Employ and Reward a Well-Experienced Administrative Staff

Take the time and effort to hire quality employees. Compensate them well—according to how well the practice is doing, not what another dentist is paying down the street. Set aside time for staff education, training, and feedback sessions.

In this day and age of working parents, consider accommodating temporary day-care emergencies. If office space permits, consider temporary day-care areas for sick or vacationing kids. If not, make arrangements with a nearby day-care center.

Utilize Your "Dentist-Extenders" Effectively

The maximal use of dental auxiliaries is crucial to a successful managed-care practice. In California, there are numerous categories recognized by the Board of Dental Examiners:

- Registered dental hygienist
- Registered dental hygienist with expanded duties
- Registered dental assistant
- Registered dental assistant with expanded duties (including coronal polish certification)

Each of these categories of dental auxiliaries is able to perform duties, some even expanded duties traditionally performed by the dentist. Recognition of these duties will allow the provider to maximize patient treatment time and increase the patient capacity of that dental facility. Dental managed-care plans keep a close eye on patient capacity and cannot assign more patients to a network provider whose patient capacity has stagnated.

Create a Working Relationship with Each Specialty Provider

Do not make the mistake of believing that since referral specialists are limited to those in a dental managed-care plan's specialty provider network, the primary care dentist simply initiates the referral and lets the dental plan take over. Remember that the PCD is also the case manager and is responsible for the coordination of care for any given patient.

Despite this responsibility, it is also good practice sense to keep in contact with specialty network providers. Dental managed-care plans will accommodate requests for referral to a specific specialist, especially one who has an excellent working relationship with the primary care dentist. As managed care grows, and more patients are transitioned from traditional plans to DMO plans, specialists have a unique opportunity to recommend that these new enrollees select certain primary care dentists whom they know and work with.

Help Patients Develop Realistic Expectations and Promote Better Oral Health

Remember—managed care rewards those providers who are health-oriented and are able to treat dental conditions in the earliest stages. Reinforce oral hygiene practices constantly and bring in the staff to support these efforts. Both dentists and staff personnel can verbally congratulate those patients who are compliant and cooperative. After all, their health is contributing to the health of the dental practice.

Closely Monitor the Financial Aspects of Each Dental Managed-Care Program

No dental practice should ignore the advantages of computerization. It is difficult to imagine any dental facility remaining competitive without some level of computer usage. Dental practice software is advancing rapidly both in user-friendliness and power. Dental practice software that does not include modules to track that portion of your practice devoted to managed care is nearly obsolete.

Examine financial records monthly for inaccuracies—they do happen. Review the monthly capitation checks on the basis of patient age and number of enrollees that you have on record and reconcile this with the plans' reporting. Again, the use of computers for these functions is crucial to cost-effective dental practices.

Successful dentists in today's marketplace maintain their practices by conserving resources, hiring qualified staff, providing training, improving professional skills through continuing education, and involving patients in treatment decisions and emphasizing their responsibility towards dental health.

CHAPTER 10

BEFORE YOU JOIN: 15 QUESTIONS YOU MUST ASK OF EVERY PLAN

"The real questions are the ones that obtrude upon your consciousness whether you like it or not, the ones that make your mind start vibrating like a jackhammer, the ones that you 'come to terms with' only to discover that they are still there. The real questions refuse to be placated. They barge into your life at the times when it seems most important for them to stay away. They are the questions asked most frequently and answered most inadequately, the ones that reveal their true natures slowly, reluctantly, most often against your will."

INGRID BENGIS (1944–), U.S. AUTHOR. "MANHATING," *COMBAT IN THE EROGENOUS ZONE* (1973) FROM *THE COLUMBIA DICTIONARY OF QUOTATIONS* (COLUMBIA UNIVERSITY PRESS, 1993).

It is fair to say that dental managed-care plans will ask many questions of you. They have questions in search of an answer, and plan representatives have learned to not be the least shy about asking.

Dentists must ask many questions as well. Indeed, as more is learned about dental managed care and its potential to radically change the way that dentistry is practiced, there are critical questions that spring to mind.

The purpose of this chapter is to focus your attention on 15 key questions that you must ask prospective plans. Each one should be answered thoroughly and unhesitatingly by each dental managed-care plan that approaches you. They may well act as springboards, causing you to jump to other questions. These questions are where you start, not where you end. Remember that both parties will and should be asking questions of each other throughout the life of the provider and plan relationship—this is the essence of communications.

THE 15 QUESTIONS

1. HOW IS MY REIMBURSEMENT TO BE DETERMINED?

Don't accept an answer as terse as "capitation" or "relative value units." Although the general industry determinants of reimbursement are discussed in detail within this book, you will want to know exactly how the dental managed-care plan intends to reimburse you.

The method that they describe to you should be replete with examples, including actual printouts of provider reimbursement data in current use. It is a simple matter for a dental plan to block out the name(s) of the dentists involved and preserve confidentiality. Some dental managed-care plans have taken a more progressive and user-friendly stance by offering videotapes, multimedia PC-based presentations, and printed tutorials; anything that will allow you to study and understand their particular spin on provider payments.

2. HOW OFTEN AM I GOING TO BE PAID?

As important as knowing how you will be paid is knowing how often you will be paid. Does the plan have adequate cash reserves in case payment problems occur between plan and purchaser, or if a government regulator should freeze payments to the plan for a brief period? These events may have never been experienced by the dental managed-care plan being queried—but financial contingencies must be in place regardless of past inexperience.

The potential provider of managed-care services would be wise to inquire as to the dental managed-care plan's financial history, especially in those states who do not require special licensure and tangible net equity (TNE) requirements to guard against insolvency. If a plan should become insolvent, the provider may still be responsible for those patients whose dental treatment is still in progress. In this eventuality, the dental managed-care plan should have purchased reinsurance specifically earmarked for provider payments.

Never accept a dental plan that tries to make capitation payments to providers only when enrollees actually complete an encounter (at least an office visit). This is known as payment on contact, and is nothing short of scandalous on the part of unscrupulous dental plans. This arrangement does not allow the provider to spread costs (and risk) among his or her assigned patients, which should represent a normal distribution of high-to-low utilizers of dental services. It is axiomatic that nonusers help to pay for users in any insurance arrangement. If an insurance company could not make a profit under a "payment on contact" situation regarding the premiums that they collect, neither can the provider make a profit under this payment scenario. Look elsewhere.

3. CAN I BILL PATIENTS FOR NONCOVERED SERVICES?

Nearly every dental managed-care plan will say yes to this question. Unfortunately, many managed-care enrollees are left with the impression that every dental service is covered. The problem really arises when you inform the patient that they require a service not covered by their dental plan's scope of benefits. Patients who are used to paying a portion of their dental care costs have an easier time understanding benefit exclusions than do their managed-care counterparts.

Patient education is the only true solution to this dilemma. Providers should carefully examine the patient's Evidence of Coverage brochure and have administrative personnel do the same. It is also incumbent upon each dental managed-care plan to not misrepresent the scope of dental services obtainable at no cost to the enrollee.

4. CAN THE PLAN CHANGE THE SCOPE OF BENEFITS UNDER ITS AGREEMENT WITH PLAN ENROLLEES WITHOUT MY CONSENT?

As unconscionable as it may be, this situation has happened (albeit infrequently). It is an area that is often overlooked by providers who, in their zeal to negotiate a satisfactory provider agreement, forget that other legal contracts govern a dental managed-care plan's business as well.

The simple answer here is that all providers in a dental plan's provider network should be told about changes in their patients' benefit structure—the sooner the better—and providers must have their reimbursements adjusted accordingly.

5. WHAT BILLING FORMS WILL BE USED?

For most providers, exasperated by the mountain of paperwork required by indemnity or fee-for-service plans, this question often brings surprisingly good news.

For the primary care dentist who receives monthly capitation payments for specified dental services, claim forms are a thing of the past. The plan will require some form of encounter data reporting (covered in depth in another chapter) in order to account for services provided, quality assurance, and utilization monitoring. This information can be collected on checklist-style forms preprinted with all provider data, or may be submitted electronically.

Specialists and out-of-network providers will still have to submit claims as precedence to payment, although here the opportunity for electronic claim submission remains a viable and welcome alternative.

6. WHO IS RESPONSIBLE FOR DETERMINING PATIENT ELIGIBILITY?

Providers should not be burdened with anything beyond a "good-faith effort" in determining a patient's eligibility. Dental managed-care plans must bear full responsibility for the issuance of plan members' identification cards that have safeguards against fraud and abuse.

In the event that a patient should arrive in the dental office without a card, then telephone authorization (with office personnel verifying the enrollee through other forms of identification) should suffice—even if the plan later declares that the patient was ineligible.

There exists a myriad of safeguards available to any and all health-care plans to ensure accurate determination of patient eligibility. If these safeguards should fail, the provider who makes a good-faith effort should never be denied payment as a result.

7. WHAT ARE THE WAYS THAT MY PARTICIPATION MAY BE TERMINATED?

No dentist ever looks forward to the day that business relations with a dental plan must cease. Even with dental managed-care plans who failed to deliver as promised, the severance of ties can be as messy as a nasty divorce.

There are two basic ways that provider termination is classified: "with cause" or "without cause." Termination of a provider "with cause" requires time invested by dental plan personnel and detailed documentation of offenses, breach of contract, or any transgressions on the part of the dentist. Termination of a provider "without cause" is as easy as invoking the clause in a provider's contract allowing for either party to terminate the agreement within a specified time frame.

Allowing either party to terminate an agreement "without cause" certainly has its place in business, for the intention was to foster cooperation and satisfaction between both parties. If one side should ever falter, then the business and legal relationship could be terminated given sufficient notice, and hopefully without the need for prolonged, expensive litigation.

The problem in our context arises when this privilege is abused by dental managed-care plans. During the First Annual Dental Managed Care Congress (held in San Francisco in early August of 1994), a panel of dental managed-care plan administrators remarked that provider termination "with cause" rarely happened. The majority of dental managed-care plan industry spokespersons present agreed that provider terminations done "without cause" were the norm.

One particular dental managed-care plan made it clear that the reason for "without cause" terminations becoming so prevalent was due to the legal and monetary issues of being taken into court if any terminated dentist disagreed with the causes. In short, this tactic is an attempt to avoid wrongful termination lawsuits.

Despite the need for dental managed-care plans to practice risk management, this is a dangerous direction for the dental managed-care industry to be moving. Invoking a contractual clause in such a fashion can be an invitation for dental plans to become sloppy and inattentive in their provider relations, quality assurance, and related functions. While it may be true that such contractual clauses are bidirectional—that is, they can be invoked by either party—the increasing use of "without cause" provider terminations is fundamentally disturbing.

For now, the dentist should ask the dental managed-care plan for data on the number of terminations over the past three years, how many were overturned on appeal, and the proportion of "with cause" versus "without cause" provider terminations. If a dental managed-care plan has operated for more than three years without a single provider termination "with cause," be suspicious of what that particular plan might do to terminate your participation.

8. WHAT ARE THE PLAN'S POLICIES FOR ALLOWING ME TO RENEGOTIATE MY PROVIDER AGREEMENT?

Try as we all must, no dentist nor dental managed-care plan has a crystal ball. The future can hold many unexpected surprises, and not all of them pleasant. There can be numerous instances in which the provider agreement that both parties signed has simply become obsolete. Previously, the possibility of a dental managed-care plan having to change the enrollees' benefit structure was discussed. In other cases, continuing to operate under the terms of the agreement may actually become damaging for one of the parties, usually the provider who is at-risk.

Dental managed-care plans, as with all businesses, will not encourage providers to renegotiate contracts. Such an action involves time, legal review, and associated fees and expenses. It is not in their best interests to throw the barn doors open in this regard.

It is extremely naive to believe that in the dynamic world of dental managed care, situations requiring amendments to existing contracts would never occur. Dental managed-care plans should have policies in place to address these situations and should not be hesitant to share these policies with the inquiring dentist. Such policies may even be explicitly stated within the provider agreements themselves.

9. HOW WILL PATIENTS BE ASSIGNED TO MY PRACTICE?

For dentists who practice in major metropolitan areas, this question is often an extremely critical one. The answer can literally decide the fate of your practice, should you decide to join a dental managed-care plan's provider network.

This question is primarily aimed at those dental managed-care plans that are of the mixed-model variety. These dental plans operate both plan-owned clinics as well as administer a provider network. This situation creates a potential for conflict within the plan—patients who are assigned to plan-owned clinics usually generate greater profit for the dental managed-care plan than if the same patient were assigned to a network provider.

Similarly, the mechanism of patient assignment may actually generate instances of adverse selection. If a patient is known to have a great need for dental treatment (from existing dental records or a plan-conducted screening exam), and such patients are sent in greater numbers to network providers than to plan-owned facilities, then adverse selection has occurred. For the provider who is at-risk for all or part of a scope of benefits, such assignment practices can destroy a dental practice.

Clearly, the dental managed-care plan must be able to ensure that patient assignments are conducted equitably. The dental plan must not conduct any internal marketing tactics that would lead a newly enrolled patient to believe that plan-owned facilities are superior to any provider's office within the network. It can be argued that in "mixed-model" dental managed-care plans, a third-party contractor should conduct all patient assignments and reassignments.

Regardless of whether a particular dental plan owns and operates clinical facilities, the mechanism of patient assignment remains a critical area that must be judged as fair and efficient by all providers participating in the network.

10. WHAT ARE THE PLAN'S POLICIES WITH REGARD TO THE USE OF DENTAL LABS?

For some dental managed-care plans, especially those recently born of companies traditionally dealing only in medical managed-care plans, this question seems trivial. As long as a blood lab, for instance, is certified and easily accessible, a medical doctor may not have any concerns about which lab(s) he or she can use for their patients.

The relationship between restorative dentists and their dental labs is a completely different story. Working relationships have been forged; quality has been judged; a comfort zone has been established, whereby the dentist knows what a particular dental lab can be entrusted to perform, and the resultant lab fees built into the fee schedule.

Some dental managed-care plans, having stumbled into the arena, have been met with howls from providers forced to "divorce" their favorite and trusted dental labs in favor of a plan-contracted (or even plan-owned) dental lab service. As a result, plans have responded with one or more of the following policies:

- If a provider uses a plan-approved dental lab, no fees are charged
- If a provider uses an independent dental lab, the provider pays the entire lab bill
- No plan-contracted dental lab exists, and the provider pays all or a portion of the lab bill

The author knows of one instance where not only is a plan-contracted dental lab available as a no-cost option to providers, but the same lab can be used for that provider's nonmanaged-care patients at a considerable discount.

There exists no single, satisfying answer to this question. Dental managed-care plans are wise to offer as many alternatives to their providers as possible—the providers, in turn, must recognize that cost containment is best achieved when the plan is able to freely negotiate in the marketplace. If a dental managed-care plan's quality assurance program is working properly, then quality control standards should be maintained at any dental lab that is made available. With an ever-increasing tendency towards vertical integration of health-care purchasers and suppliers, plan-owned dental labs are becoming more commonplace.

11. HOW DOES THE PLAN DECIDE ON A PROVIDER'S MAXIMUM PATIENT CAPACITY?

Just as critical as the question concerning patient assignment is this corollary to it. Great harm can come to the provider expecting to receive 500 new patients from a dental managed-care plan, only to find that his or her "capacity" will only allow for the assignment of 50 patients at the present time.

For some states (California in particular), there exist regulations that establish maximum provider-to-patient ratios for primary care providers. These ratios are often devised with medical models in mind and are applied to allied health professions without modification. In

California's Knox-Keene Dental Guidelines (see Appendix I), there exists a maximum ratio of one provider for every 2,000 patients, or higher if the managed-care plan can demonstrate an alternative mechanism acceptable to state regulators.

The American Dental Association does not support the use of arbitrary ratios for the determination of maximum patient capacity.[27] The ADA recognizes that dynamic mechanisms and monitoring systems must be in place and consistently applied to the entire provider network.

For the time being, it is imperative that a dental managed-care plan demonstrate a well-planned (perhaps time-tested) method for the determination of provider capacity. Providers should know what staff positions can be considered as "extenders," allowing for the assignment of more patients to their offices. Conversely, dental managed-care plans cannot merely wait for a provider to scream "enough!" as the signal to close an office to future patients.

12. HOW DOES THE PLAN'S INTERNAL PEER REVIEW SYSTEM WORK?

Most dentists in practice today are familiar with the peer review systems in place with organized dental associations. Much of what is currently in place throughout the United States stems from the pioneering work of the California Dental Association.

In the best managed-care plans, peer review provides opportunities for network providers to involve themselves in quality oriented activities. As an important subset of a complete quality assurance program, peer review offers more than just dentists judging dentists. It should also offer providers a way to better understand the dynamics of dental managed care and allow peer review committees to provide feedback to the plan's administration.

Beware those dental plans with static memberships on peer review committees, or those staffed completely by plan-employed dentists. Likewise, the actions, decisions, and workings of any peer review group should not be alien to those already established by the dental profession.

The Health Care Quality Improvement Act of 1986, while aimed primarily towards medicine, has important applications in dental managed care. The act established the National Practitioner Data Bank and gave additional direction to peer review groups. Every dental managed-care plan needs to be fully cognizant of the act and its implications on dental plan operations, peer review activities, and reporting requirements.

Knowing how a dental managed-care plan's peer review system works is vital as dentistry enters into a new age of accountability, with national report cards on both providers and plans being discussed, and increasing insistence by purchasers that dental managed-care plans assure quality dental care.

13. WHAT ARE MY RIGHTS IN REGARD TO INSPECTING ANY PLAN RECORDS PERTAINING TO MY PRACTICE?

Even though many documents held by a dental managed-care plan can be deemed confidential or proprietary with restricted access, each and every network provider must know how he or she stands with the plan, financially and otherwise.

Few dentists will take the time to physically inspect the plan's records at its place of business, but reasonable access should be granted nonetheless. Providers should be prepared to pay for the duplication costs if a large number of documents are requested.

Providers have the right to accurate information about their participation in a managed-care plan, just as much as the plan has the right to accurate information (i.e., encounter data) concerning patient care.

The more progressive dental managed-care plans will use their management information systems (MIS) to its full potential, sharing information with plan providers in order to educate them and improve dental practices.

14. HOW DOES THE PLAN HANDLE COMPLAINTS, GRIEVANCES, AND APPEALS FROM PROVIDERS?

Dental managed-care plans must have policies and procedures to track, monitor, and resolve problems brought to their attention by providers. Timeliness is an important issue in this process—the longer it takes to achieve problem resolution, the less chance it has of being mutually satisfying to plan and providers.

A poorly functioning provider grievance system may be the result of:

- An intrinsically poor system design
- An inordinately high number of provider complaints
- Obstinacy on the part of the dental managed-care plan to achieve resolutions

Every dental managed-care plan in every state should fall under the regulatory auspices of a specific state agency. In California, the Department of Corporations is the legally empowered agency for health plan licensure and monitoring. In other states, the duty may belong to insurance commissioners. The provider must know what will happen if problem resolution cannot be achieved by the plan—does the matter simply die, or can the appeal be elevated to the regulatory (state) level?

Most states have provided for patient appeals and "fair hearing" processes involving administrative law judges but have not followed suit in providing such avenues for providers. This situation may change with the growth of dental managed care and the evolution of health-care reform nationally.

The better dental plans will build grievance processes that result in positive outcomes for the vast majority of provider complaints. Prospective providers would be well advised to communicate with colleagues already in the provider network about their experiences.

15. DOES THE PLAN PROVIDE FOR ANY EXTERNAL (THIRD-PARTY) AUDITS OF ITS QUALITY ASSURANCE PROGRAM?

Audits performed by recognized entities or companies not affiliated in any manner with a dental managed-care plan are becoming increasingly important. While most shareholders are aware of federal requirements for independent accounting audits of publicly held companies, few dental patients think about applying the same process to quality assurance programs.

Quality assurance programs, as discussed in chapter 5, are essential to the successful operation of any dental managed-care plan. Whether required by government regulations or not, managed-care plans should view these independent audits as annual tune-ups for their QA activities. In addition, having a recent, successful audit on the record can be a tremendous marketing tool for drawing new patients, purchasers, and providers into the dental managed-care plan.

In summary, dentists should never shrink away from asking these or other questions of a dental managed-care plan. Successful plans have nothing to hide and view such interest from a prospective provider as a positive sign that further communications will be time well spent.

CHAPTER 11

PROVIDER AGREEMENTS— MAKING THE DECISION

*"Money is better than poverty,
if only for financial reasons."*
WOODY ALLEN (1935–), U.S. FILMMAKER.
"THE EARLY ESSAYS," *WITHOUT FEATHERS* (1976)
FROM *THE COLUMBIA DICTIONARY OF QUOTATIONS*
(COLUMBIA UNIVERSITY PRESS, 1993).

Agreeing to become a part of a dental managed-care plan's provider network is not simply a matter of contract negotiation. It is a critical decision that involves a great deal of homework by the dentist before reaching a conclusion. Making the right choices is crucial to professional survival—it can even dramatically affect the value of your entire practice when the time comes to sell. There is a myriad of complexities to be found in provider agreements and subcontracts, and understanding them usually requires more than this chapter can adequately relate.

Before delving into the subject matter, a word to the wise—prior to signing any provider agreement, have it reviewed by a contracts attorney with experience in health-care issues. Yes, the American Dental Association does offer a contract analysis service, but their function is more to explain individual clauses within the contract than to advise you about the ramifications of signing it. Even the ADA recommends the advice of trained counsel and the use of a practice management consultant with experience in managed care. Also keep in mind that this is a negotiating process—if you object to any contract clause, select alternate language and communicate it to the plan. Dental plans commonly use boilerplate contracts and are not opposed to making reasonable changes to them, including entering into a process of offers and counteroffers. Pay special attention to the small changes that add up. Having the monthly capitation payment per patient increased by 1%, cutting payment cycles by 25%, or shifting one or two higher cost procedures from the category covered by the capitation fee into one that allows for patient co-payments—these actions and others can make a large improvement in a provider's total compensation.

Any provider agreement that you are offered from a dental plan will be tied to a benefit agreement (see Appendix II). This other agreement is essentially what the dental plan and purchaser have mutually agreed to in terms of benefit levels, co-payments, and the like. The term will undoubtedly appear several times in any provider agreement; since it obligates you contractually as well as the dental plan itself, the benefit agreement should be open to inspection by you and your attorney upon request. In addition, you should know what the dental managed-care plan intends to do should the benefit agreement be modified—or you could end up providing additional dental services without an appropriate increase in reimbursement to offset the changes.

REIMBURSEMENT

This will undoubtedly be one of the first areas that you review. It will provide you with the information that you will need to compare this plan to others that you have or might be contracting with (see Chapter 12, Fractional Practice Analysis).

You may be pleasantly surprised that dental managed-care reimbursements are not simply monthly capitation checks, where you receive X dollars per patient per month for those patients assigned to your office. This "straight capitation" reimbursement placed too much risk on the dentist and has largely been augmented with other payment incentives. Capitation remains the primary method of provider reimbursement in dental managed care—the other situations are either incentives or alternatives to it. The chart on the following page illustrates the payment methods used for HMO-based primary care physicians (see Fig. 11–1). Dentistry is reaching a similar complexity.

Herb Kaufman, regional dental director for CIGNA Western Region, points out that besides the monthly capitation check, compensation to

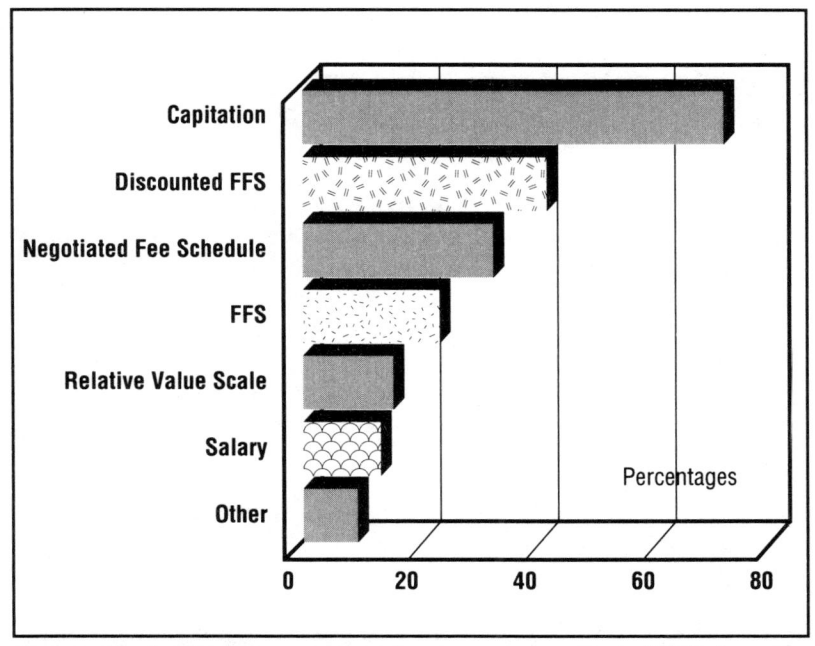

Figure 11–1. Primary care physicians' payment methods (HMO-based) [Source: The Interstudy Competitive Edge, (Group Health Insurance Association of America, 1991)]

providers can take other forms, including member co-payments, supplemental payments, and visit fees. According to Dr. Kaufman, "If capitation is the only source of revenue to providers for all needed care, there's a risk situation for the provider. They're being asked to provide care for a population with an unknown dental need, yet they receive a fixed monthly revenue to provide that care. The dentist has to feel that the compensation mechanism is just and equitable. Once that occurs, the level of service is commensurate with the fee-for-service marketplace."[28]

The prospective dental managed-care provider will need to be sensitive to the issue of "withholds" or "pool funds." This is an area in which a certain amount of providers' reimbursements are held in a special account used for contingencies, referral costs, etc. The dental managed-care plan must be clear about the exact amount that each provider will contribute, how the account is monitored, and how often reconciliation occurs. Some plans tie the return of pool funds to each individual provider's quality and efficacy; others tie it to the aggregate performance of the entire provider network. Try to negotiate for the former, because the latter leaves you vulnerable to the actions of dentists you cannot control.

Just as important as knowing what the plan will pay you for is knowing what the patient will pay you for. This distinction is easily clouded in many contracts. Pay close attention to the following terms:

Covered Dental Services. This simply means all of the benefits that the dental plan and purchaser agreed to in the benefit agreement. It tells you nothing about how a specific service is to be paid.

Principal Benefits with Co-payments. These procedures involve patient payments, and you must make the effort to collect.

Principal Benefits without Co-payments. These are often called the "straight capitation" services, for they involve no out-of-pocket expense to the patient. Accordingly, these procedures are performed at-risk by the dentist, and the utilization by patients of this subset of dental benefits will directly impact the profitability of a provider's practice.

Principal Excluded Procedures and Services. Use caution here. Many plans will tell you that it is all right to "upsell" a patient on an excluded service, because then you may charge them directly for that service.

Technically, this is true, but only after the dentist has presented the patient with *all acceptable alternative treatment options*. If the managed-care patient then decides to receive an excluded service, the provider must fully document this decision including the alternatives discussed.

Principal Limitations. These are procedures that are a benefit, but with specific time restrictions (once every year, adult teeth only, etc.). Don't confuse these with exclusions.

These hybrid forms of reimbursement should be clearly and accurately spelled out in the provider agreement. Do not hesitate to seek the advice of an accountant and ask the dental plan's provider relations staff to help explain them. If the dental managed-care plan's own staff cannot interpret their own payment methods, a warning bell should sound.

16 ELEMENTS OF SPECIAL IMPORTANCE IN A PROVIDER AGREEMENT/CONTRACT

1. TERMS AND CONDITIONS (AND TERMINATION)

The contract should have a definite date of expiration, including conditions whereby both the dentist and the dental plan may terminate the agreement. Like divorcing one's spouse, the differences between terminating a contract "without cause" or "with cause" can wreak havoc on a dental practice unless they are spelled out clearly.

In order to capture the largest number of enrolled patients, and have sufficient time to bring them into a maintenance phase, aim for a provider agreement with a term of two years minimum, with annual automatic renewal for an additional three years. These terms are identical to what the dental benefits industry strives to attain in its own contracts with purchasers.

Pay very special attention to any clauses dealing with "treatment in progress." Some dental plans have interpreted this very broadly to mean that the dentist is responsible for completing the entire treatment plan after termination from the program. More reasonable dental managed-care plans interpret the clause to mean that any procedure already started (i.e., endodontic therapy on #20) must be completed. In the dentist's favor is when the agreement allows him to charge the patient his UCR fees for this remaining treatment, including any future treatment if the patient elects to remain at that office. Do not place yourself in the position of being prevented from charging the patient, receiving no reimbursement from the dental plan and still remaining liable for that patient's continued treatment. Many dentists have found themselves in this no-win situation.

2. FUTURE MODIFICATIONS OF CONTRACT

Things change, even for the best dental plans. Nearly all will want clauses allowing them to renegotiate with the dentist under certain contingencies. Others may want the right to make unilateral changes to the contract at the sole discretion of the dental plan. These situations can be quite complex and difficult to understand. Seek legal advice and remember—you may wish to renegotiate the contract for reasons of your own, and an attorney can suggest the appropriate modifications.

3. HOLD HARMLESS CLAUSES

Thankfully, the traditional "hold harmless" clause is virtually extinct. Particularly in the world of dental managed care, a dental plan cannot absolve itself of all wrongdoing by shifting liability onto the shoulders of the provider. If one appears in a contract presented to you, ask that it be removed. Your attorney can give you numerous legal case citations in which the courts have failed to uphold them.

4. REFERRALS

These sections can be amalgamations of both the referral policies and procedures of a plan as well as contractual "withholds," in which the dental plan holds back a portion of every PCD's payment for a reserve fund intended to pay for specialty care. There is nothing inherently wrong with this situation, providing that mechanisms exist for dividing up any excess moneys in reserve on a regular (usually annual) basis.

One situation that should be avoided at all costs is when the plan places the PCD at complete financial risk for all specialty referrals. Fortunately, this situation is seen in very few contracts. If you find it in your provider agreement, get it changed, or simply look elsewhere.

With respect to the dental plan's referral protocols, ensure that they are reasonable and allow for all dentally necessary referrals to be made, with any denials subject to an appeals process. Remember that the courts have made it very clear that the dentist cannot compromise the treatment plan or dental health of a patient due to any contractual limitations of that patient's dental benefits.

5. UTILIZATION REVIEW

Yes, you will be subject to periodic reviews of the utilization of services for your assigned patients. You will also be asked to participate in peer review activities towards this purpose with your colleagues. This is an integral and necessary part of a dental managed-care plan's quality assurance program. It should be sophisticated enough to be virtually transparent to your day-to-day practice. Should an audit team come calling, however, the situation is likely to be more educational than punitive. This is how the best dental managed-care plans keep their providers satisfied.

6. GRIEVANCE SYSTEM

Just as your patients will want a way to air out their grievances, so will you. There should be a way to file a grievance with a plan, including an appeals process. Yes, you can always complain to governmental agencies and the like, or even take the plan to court. These options are time-consuming, expensive, and unnecessary when dealing with a reasonable managed-care plan. Both the provider agreement and plan manuals should support an equitable grievance system.

7. ARBITRATION

This is becoming commonplace in nearly all business contracts today, for the simple reason that no one enjoys going to court. Expect that it will be part of every provider agreement, and your attorney can advise you as to whether it stipulates a reasonable method of dispute resolution.

8. INSURANCE

The dental managed-care plan will be concerned with the amount of professional liability insurance that you carry and will always set minimum limits. Additionally, proof of insurance (usually your policy's declarations page) is a standard request.

If the company objects to your insurance carrier, it might be for good reason. Have the dental plan explain their objection—you might find a better carrier as a result.

9. MOST-FAVORED NATION CLAUSE

Increasingly, fee-for-service plans have used this clause to secure the lowest fees for their plan members. Briefly, it requires you to give the plan's members the lowest fee that you would charge to any patient, perhaps through another dental plan's contract. Managed-care plans will carry this clause as well if member co-payments and other allowable patient charges are made.

Although this clause is certainly not popular with dentists, its use and enforcement by plans is increasing. Bottom line—be careful about which patient group or plan you give your greatest discount to, lest you be forced contractually to give that discount to every patient that enters your office.

10. NONCOMPETITION CLAUSES

As with the "hold harmless" clause, these clauses have not been having good days in courtrooms recently. Since they attempt to limit your ability to participate in other programs, they have run afoul of a number of laws and may be unenforceable. It is doubtful whether one would even appear on a recently drafted provider agreement.

11. ASSIGNMENT AND/OR DELEGATION

Many dentists intend to have the capitation portion of their practice handled by an associate. This clause may prevent such a situation, with the dental managed-care plan fully expecting the contracting provider to be the treating provider as well. If this is part of your practice strategy, carefully examine your rights to delegate treatment responsibilities to an associate dentist.

By the same right, the dental managed-care plan that contracted with you might be sold to another plan. This consolidation of the health-care market is happening with increasing regularity. If the provider agreement does not discuss such an eventuality, you might consider raising the issue. Life under the new plan might be just fine, or the contract might require termination and the negotiation of new provider agreements under different terms and conditions than you had anticipated.

12. LIQUIDATED DAMAGES

Rather than go to court and have a judge and jury decide on damage awards, many businesses prefer to predetermine the amount of damages owed by both parties at the outset—namely, within the body of a contract. In provider agreements, however, most of the obligations belong to the dentist. The dentist, then, would owe considerable moneys to the dental managed-care plan should any breach of contract occur. The odds are stacked against the provider in nearly all possible scenarios.

The American Dental Association's contract analysis service advises dentists *never* to agree to liquidated damages without the advice of counsel.

13. AGREEING TO ABIDE BY THE PLAN'S RULES, REGULATIONS, AND PROCEDURES

It is not unreasonable for any dental managed-care plan to ask its providers to play by the rules. It *is* unreasonable to ask them to play and make the rulebook unavailable. Ask to have the rules spelled out right in the contract. If this is too unwieldy, then have the rulebook or plan policy manual incorporated into the contract by reference, including the full title and date of issuance.

14. STATE OF JURISDICTION FOR DISPUTES

This becomes a concern only if the dental managed-care plan is headquartered in another state from where you practice. If in the eventuality of a legal action, you must appear in their state, then the costs associated with this situation will become staggering. Try to get jurisdiction within your own state.

15. RISK POOLS, WITHHOLDS, AND BONUS PAYMENTS

Get the contract to specify the size of the pooled accounts, which providers are included, how much money will go into the account, when contributions are made, and when pool funds will be returned. Do the same for bonus payments. If the language here is unclear, dental plans may be using such funds to cover administrative shortfalls. In essence, you are providing the dental plan with an interest-free loan.

16. STOP-LOSS ARRANGEMENTS

Whether the cause is adverse selection or poor patient assignment and the like, any reason beyond a prudent provider's control that threatens his or her financial viability should be subject to a stop-loss arrangement. In these cases, the dental managed-care plan will ensure that the provider's financial risk ends, and operational costs are covered until the situation is resolved.

Provider agreements or subcontracts are necessary rites of passage into any dental managed-care provider network. Never sign one until you are completely comfortable with its content and *always* seek the advice of experienced legal counsel. Appendix II has a sample provider agreement that, while created as a generic document, is similar to current provider agreements used by dental plans. Study Appendix II carefully and decide how you would evaluate the agreement.

CHAPTER 12

FRACTIONAL PRACTICE ANALYSIS

"I have always thought that one man of tolerable abilities may work great changes, and accomplish great affairs among mankind, if he first forms a good plan, and, cutting off all amusements or other employments that would divert his attention, make the execution of that same plan his sole study and business."

BENJAMIN FRANKLIN (1706–90), U.S. STATESMAN, WRITER. *AUTOBIOGRAPHY* (1868) FROM *THE COLUMBIA DICTIONARY OF QUOTATIONS* (COLUMBIA UNIVERSITY PRESS, 1993)

This chapter deals with overcoming a common failing of dentists in private practice—failing to know what is happening to their business. William Pollock, FSA, had these comments concerning one's success in managed care:

What often separates winners from losers under capitation is that winners do their homework, develop a plan, and monitor its execution. Specifically, successful groups are taking the following steps:

- Perform due diligence up front
- Know their current dental efficiency strengths and weaknesses
- Develop treatment guidelines or protocols consistent with their definition of dental efficiency
- Establish performance targets
- Make sure either they or their managed-care partner can provide proper data to monitor results
- Monitor results, taking corrective actions when necessary.[29]

Those plans that are successful in the managed-care arena will be held to levels of accountability never before required under fee-for-service. The individual dentist, the largest percentage of whom are in private practice, must hold himself/herself fully accountable as well.

Fractional practice analysis is merely a method of keeping you on track. It can be thought of as a natural extension of proper business accounting in a dental office environment. The small degree of complexity that is added to one's practice is vastly offset by the increased degree of control, and concomitant analysis, that it offers. Fractional practice analysis allows the provider of care to monitor and measure the performance characteristics of each dental benefit program (each of them a fraction of your total practice) that can either contribute to or degrade his or her practice income.

It is intriguing to note at this point that among our medical colleagues, a variety of reimbursement mechanisms currently exists within medical HMOs. Capitation is the predominant method of reimbursement but is not the only method. That is why it is vital that dentists do not equate capitation with managed care. One is a payment mechanism; the other is an alternative health-care delivery system.

It chagrins many purchasers of health-care benefits, most of them businesses themselves, that dentists traditionally have not followed pricing methodologies when setting fees. All too often, fees are determined by either: (1) what the FFS plan will accept upon filing a fee schedule, or (2) what a colleague in the area charges for similar dental procedures. Some dental-practice managers argue that it may be unrealistic to expect dentists to determine their own fees.

Richard Ryan, president of Dental Management Decisions, recently wrote:

> *It is an awesome responsibility, possibly even an unrealistic responsibility, to ask a dentist or physician to set "reasonable" fees for his or her services. What defines reasonable? What makes a crown worth $500, $600, or $700?*
>
> *How have crown fees historically been established? Were these fees set by some scientific or calculated financial-pricing formula? Or, has it more to do with what other dentists down the street were charging and/or how high of a fee Delta would allow you to file? If there were any scientific approach to fee structuring, do you really think that a crown would have a $500 fee while a four-surface amalgam has a $100 (or less) fee?*[30]

Now that dentistry is facing market pressures that other industries have faced for many years, purchasers (and dental plans) are no longer willing to tolerate escalating fees based on nonexistent pricing methods.

It is a natural reaction for dentists to become defensive at this point. They point out that the costs of OSHA compliance, materials, labor costs, etc., are very clearly known—and many can quote you their office overhead costs quite readily.

The problem is this: there is no such thing as indefinite fixed costs. Any and all costs incurred in business can potentially be altered. Rent too high? Renegotiate one's lease or relocate. Staff salaries seem to be a formidable expense? Reorganize staff duties and/or hours within your office. Every business in America faces decisions on costs that impact success or failure. In our world of dental practice, we must know if the dental benefit programs in which we participate influence our interests either positively or negatively.

Relative Value Unit (RVU)

Attempts have been made to develop time- and resource-based methods by which to set a fair market value on professional services. In the relative value unit (RVU) concept, a dental plan will develop a set of unit values correlating to common ADA procedure codes.

Each single unit represents 15 minutes of chair time expended by a general dentist. This method presumes the availability of a full-time dental assistant and two fully equipped operatories per dentist. The dental hygienist's time is valued at one-third of the dentist, and any services that could be performed by the hygienist (even if performed by a dentist) are valued at the lower rate. The dental assistant's time is not considered an independent factor, as these assisting costs are included in the cost of the dentist's time (assuming that four-handed dentistry is the current dental practice norm).

Different dental plans have altered the manner in which RVUs are computed and used in actual practice. Accordingly, many different versions have appeared.

For the practicing dentist, the RVU provides an important benchmark. Using similar analytic patterns, one can determine the cost of treating an average patient per chair hour. In certain plans, reimbursement to the dentist is heavily marketed around this "chair-hour cost." A common rationale for participation is that the plan will send patients to fill in unused chair time. Compensation to the dentist can then appear reduced from FFS levels (since overhead costs have already been incurred) without a real loss of FFS equivalency. Less money is better than no money.

Fractional Practice Analysis

FPA is a totally by-the-numbers approach to separately analyzing the various dental plan contributions to a dental practice. For this reason, it is important to note that the resultant analysis will only be as accurate as the financial data used to derive it.

Table 12–1 shows the breakdown of costs versus revenue for a hypothetical dental practice, this one owned by Dr. M.C., for the month of July 1994.

Table 12-1
Breakdown of Costs vs. Revenue.

Statement of Income, M.C., D.D.S., July 1994	Percentage of Gross Income	Amount (in dollars)
INCOME		
Production	100%	60,000
Collections	95%	57,000
EXPENSES		
Salaries	18%	10,800
Advertising	1%	600
Insurance	2%	1,200
Employee benefits	3%	1,800
Communications	2%	1,200
Expenses relating to collections	1%	600
Office supplies	5%	3,000
Rent, utilities	6%	3,600
Professional supplies	9%	5,400
Lab expenses	6%	3,600
Payroll taxes	3%	1,800
Miscellaneous	1%	600
Total expenses	1–51%	34,200

The next step is crucial, because the dentist must know the source of patients by plan, in addition to that group's contribution to the practice. The next step of FPA is seen in Table 12–2.

Table 12–2
Source of Patients by Contributing Plans.

Plan	RVUs Reported	Patient Utilization	Office Visits
FFS & Cash	300	21%	55
A	587	41%	150
B	97	7%	28
C	118	8%	38
D	110	8%	33
E	148	10%	43
F	35	3%	16
G	40	3%	14
TOTAL	1,435	100%	377

Note that patient utilization is the result of dividing each plan's RVU total by the total RVU for all plans. Also note that plans A through G represent managed-care plans that are using the capitation method of payment to Dr. M.C.

Now we calculate the actual cost per RVU in Dr. M.C.'s practice for the month of July 1994, as his practice overhead divided by the total RVUs. This comes to $24. The cost per patient visit is derived similarly and is found to be $91.

Using gross income figures (actual collections), we find an income for the month of $40 per RVU and $151 per visit. Substituting net income figures, we arrive at $15 per RVU and $56 per visit.

Remember that these are only statistics and must be correlated to the actual income derived from each dental plan (see Table 12–3).

Table 12–3
Income Arrayed from All Plans.

Plan	Plan Income (dollars)	Income/RVU (dollars)	Income/Visit (dollars)
FFS & Cash	12,000	40	213
A	18,000	30	114
B	3,000	26	103
C	2,500	21	64
D	2,000	22	72
E	4,000	26	90
F	1,400	41	89
G	1,401	37	104

Previously, in calculating the cost per RVU and cost per patient visit, we were actually determining the break-even points for Dr. M.C.'s practice. Those figures were $25 and $95, respectively. As we review the list above, any plan's income contribution to the practice that falls below any or all of the break-even points is obviously losing money for Dr. M.C. As is evident in Table 12–3, some of the managed-care plans are not generating revenue. This is not, however, immediate grounds for Dr. M.C. to terminate his participation in these plans. Intangibles, such as patient referrals, turnover of patients into better-paying plans, etc., cannot be analyzed in these types of reports but should be considered before reaching a final conclusion.

The first step is for Dr. M.C. to revisit his understanding of the plan's benefit structure. It is not unusual to find that if a dental

Table 12-4
Fractional Practice Analysis Worksheet.

Month of _____, _____

1. Total Operating Costs _____

2. Total Collections _____

3. Total Office Visits _____

Table of Plan Contributions to Income

Plan	Capitation and incentives	Co-payments and non-benefit treatments	Number of office visits
A	B	C	D

5. Cost per visit (1 divided by 3) _____

6. Income per visit (2 divided by 3) _____

Analysis of Managed Care Plan:

B + C = Q

Q / D = Income per visit for respective plan

A comparison of item #5 to the above computation will yield the break-even point.

This form is copyrighted to Dental Management Decisions and is reprinted with permission of Dental Management Decisions.

---

managed-care plan is fully understood by both dentist and patient, and treatment plans are based on appropriate, necessary therapy, then the co-payment income may represent as much as 80% of the capitation income for an office with a sizable population of assigned managed-care patients.

Remember that this is managed care for dentistry, and that excellent communication between plans and their provider networks will become the hallmark for any successful plan. Use of the fractional practice analysis is meant to provide feedback and resolution of problems and not to promote the contractual equivalent of the OK Corral. The results of your fractional practice analysis can be the starting point for frank discussions with a dental managed-care plan that can yield positive changes.

There is a more somber note to managed care, especially for the solo practitioner who has not proactively joined an IPA or other group entity. Most managed-care programs prefer one-stop shopping for their members. They are also focused upon volume—the smallest functional provider network possible, with maximum assignment of patients to each office. Staff-model offices can perform these tasks rather easily, since their practice pattern was developed with these elements in mind. It is difficult under these circumstances for the solo practice to compete and still retain his or her existing FFS patients.

Despite these situations, no health professional should ignore a practice analysis. The fractional practice analysis worksheet contained in this book should be liberally used by all providers of dental managed care (see Table 12–4).

Chapter 13

Dropouts—Dealing with Termination from a Dental Managed-Care Program

"In an expanding universe, time is on the side of the outcast. Those who once inhabited the suburbs of human contempt find that without changing their address they eventually live in the metropolis."

QUENTIN CRISP (1908–), BRITISH AUTHOR. *THE NAKED CIVIL SERVANT* (1968) FROM *THE COLUMBIA DICTIONARY OF QUOTATIONS* (COLUMBIA UNIVERSITY PRESS, 1993).

Our medical colleagues, who have dealt with managed-care systems for many more years and with greater intensity than have their dental brethren, have found that in some areas of the country they are being terminated from their provider networks without cause.

Previously, we discussed this possibility in dental managed care, including the remarks of some industry representatives. The subject deserves its own chapter, for the seed for "termination without cause" is present in nearly every dental managed-care provider agreement (contract).

Providers who rely on a single managed-care plan for a substantial majority of their patients are particularly vulnerable to this form of termination. It is entirely possible then, if such a practice had 40% of its income derived from participation in the provider network of a single plan, to literally lose 40% of the practice after 30 days' notice (a standard feature in most termination clauses).

As the free market and mergers within the health-care industry occur, many managed-care plans find themselves having to make adjustments in their provider networks. Even if the dental plan had stellar relationships with its providers, the mere introduction of a strong competitor into the same service area coupled with the loss of key purchasers would be adequate economic incentive to downsize a provider network.

Five Ways That Dentists Can Avoid Termination

1. TRY TO GET ANY "TERMINATION WITHOUT CAUSE" LANGUAGE REMOVED FROM THE PROVIDER AGREEMENT

Good luck. It seems as if these clauses are among those that dental managed-care plans are adamant about keeping. After all, these clauses are bilateral, allowing the provider to terminate the plan under the same time constraints.

The best recommendation at this time is to get written documentation from the dental managed-care plan that the clause is strictly non-negotiable. This is a protective measure that gambles on the future—courts may rule that an "illegal contract of adhesion" has occurred if the dentist had no power to modify it.

2. PAY CLOSE ATTENTION TO THE PLAN'S CRITERIA FOR EVALUATING YOUR PERFORMANCE

Don't find yourself voted "provider of the year" one day and dropped from the network the next. You have learned enough from this book to know that every dental provider must be aware of quality assurance judgments and utilization review decisions—record and file each and every one of them that you receive. Do not allow more than 30 days to pass before you make inquiries into unusual findings or communications from the dental managed-care plan. Ask for clarification if you do not understand them. Send a written explanation on any case in which the dental managed-care plan makes inappropriate care an issue.

3. STRIVE FOR A MIXTURE OF DENTAL PROGRAMS IN YOUR PRACTICE

As attractive as some "exclusive provider arrangements" may seem, they make you into a one-trick pony. Nothing lasts forever—diversification is safer for the dentist who is new to managed care. Keep track of the performance of each part (or fraction) of your practice's sources of patients through methods like this book's fractional practice analysis.

4. NETWORK WITH THE MAJOR EMPLOYERS OF YOUR PATIENTS

Keep in contact with your patients' benefits managers. Offer to speak to employee groups on dental health topics, or set up a dental health fair. Get the dental managed-care plan to underwrite it. Managed care companies will usually consult with their major customers before terminating a dentist from the network.

5. USE YOUR INDEPENDENT PRACTICE ASSOCIATION TO EASE THE PAIN

If you are terminated, but part of an IPA, then former patients will find it easier to keep seeing you. In addition, the association may be able to wield enough collective bargaining power to keep you in the network. IPAs are by no means foolproof—but they offer distinct advantages over directly contracting with dental plans when sticky situations (like termination) arise.

DEALING WITH TERMINATION

If you find yourself terminated from the provider network, write a letter to the dental managed-care plan ASAP and ask for:

- A detailed explanation for the termination
- Copies of all documents used in making the decision, including names of individuals who were in the decision-making process
- Copies of the criteria used in making the decision to terminate
- An audience with the plan's dental director

Use any and all of this information to make a case for reinstatement. Remember that the "weakest link" in any provider termination process deals with the criteria used, which is one reason why so many dental managed-care plans prefer to terminate without cause. Getting your patients to write letters to their employers can help tremendously.

And finally, as the absolute last resort, consider litigation. Use an attorney who has had extensive experience in the health-care field, be prepared for hefty legal expenses, and gather substantial documentation to prove your case.

Rather than becoming paranoid over possible termination, providers should work to understand the markets in their area and follow the fortunes (or misfortunes) of the dental managed-care plans with which they deal. Provider networks are a precious part of dental managed care—a wise plan will only consider provider terminations when drastic market forces demand it.

Chapter 14

A Final Word

"By its very nature, the novel indicates that we are becoming. There is no final solution. There is no last word."

CARLOS FUENTES (1928–) MEXICAN NOVELIST, SHORT-STORY WRITER. *GUARDIAN* (LONDON, 24 FEBRUARY 1989).

Throughout the debates, concerns, outrage, and celebration about dental managed care, I have often found myself pitted against organized dentistry. It surprises many of my colleagues to discover that I belong (and pay dues) to the Sacramento District Dental Society, California Dental Association, American Dental Association, American Academy of Periodontology, American Board of Periodontology, and the American Board of Quality Assurance and Utilization Review Physicians.

It would be a sin for me to paint organized dentistry in any other light than what is deserved—they are largely grand organizations, well intentioned, and their leaders and members have taught the citizenry of

A Final Word

the United States more about what it takes to be dentally healthy than any managed-care plan could ever achieve.

It does, however, cause me great disappointment when I read the following, quoted from the American Dental Association: "The concept of 'managed care' has been universally promoted as a method of containing health-care costs. This system is purely cost-driven and, contrary to its title (managed care), does not concern itself with type, appropriateness, timeliness, or quality of care."[31]

It is my fervent hope that you, the dentist-reader, will consider the various aspects of dental managed care as presented in this book and draw your own conclusions. As for myself, the world of dental managed care is exciting, invigorating, and not without challenge. I would not change my involvement in it one iota. I am proud of my profession— and of being a dentist.

Sometimes, the world makes it difficult for each of us to see the importance of dentistry. Othertimes, the world allows others to see it for us. I leave you with this observation from a British colleague:

> *How about, for a change, a tale of health care triumphant in the United States? Rare though this success story is, lessons can surely by learned from it. The reason the success has gone uncelebrated may be because it concerns dental health and dentistry. Both are routinely caricatured in popular culture, particularly in television comedy, which evokes laughter by equating dental treatment with the ultimate in pain. The root canal, usually treated with little discomfort, remains enshrined in the cliché hall of fame as being synonymous with torture.*
>
> *Dental care in the United States has achieved a hallmark of success that continues to elude most areas of medical practice—economic stagnation, even decline, because of preventive measures that decisively reduce the need for many services. But when needed, those services are provided with increasing efficiency and little discomfort. One measure of success is the fading economic attractiveness of dentistry as a career. While medical school enrollments have weathered the*

> *recession almost unchanged at about 16,000 admissions per year, dental enrollments have been shrinking. Several dental schools have even shut down. In a counter-Marxian tour de force, the dental profession is tending towards putting itself out of business.*
>
> *This report on success against dental disease—surely one of humanity's greatest miseries—has come and gone with virtually no public attention. Strange how one of the finest accomplishments of health care goes uncelebrated in this health-obsessed country.*[32]

Managed care is the movement of dentistry away from disease orientation towards health orientation. Once we all become "obsessed" with healthy outcomes, and are fairly compensated for maintaining them, the world will be ready to celebrate with us.

Bryan Quattlebaum, D.D.S.

APPENDIX I

THE KNOX-KEENE DENTAL GUIDELINES

PREFACE

In the early 1970s, prepaid health plans (PHPs) had a sullied reputation. Flagrant marketing abuses, questionable quality of care, and poor access to health services were encountered in both commercial and publicly contracted programs.

In 1975, the Knox-Keene Health Care Service Plan Act (Knox-Keene) was enacted in the state of California. Knox-Keene made the California Department of Corporations the legally designated state regulatory agency for PHPs and set state licensing requirements and standards for all PHPs.

In 1985, the Department of Corporations developed what is now known as the "Knox-Keene Dental Guidelines." Although the guidelines are not all-inclusive, they were the first serious attempt at establishing standards for dental benefit plans operating within the state of California. The guidelines consist of two parts:

> Section 1: Regulations in guideline format drawn from the original Knox-Keene Act

Section 2: Quality of care guidelines (drafted with the assistance of the California Dental Association)

Section 1 remains viable to this day and will give the reader valuable insight into what managed-care dental plans are required to follow (as well as their provider network) in day-to-day operations. Section 2 is philosophically similar to *Quality Evaluation for Dental Care: Guidelines for the Assessment of Clinical Quality and Professional Performance*, published by the California Dental Association (1977). These guidelines deal primarily with the technical quality of dentistry and do not fully satisfy the complete quality assurance program needs of a dental managed-care plan. The various parameters of care established by some dental specialty organizations and the long-awaited American Dental Association's parameters of care will be more appropriate.

Keep in mind as you read these guidelines that any regulations made after 1985, especially in regard to OSHA and the Board of Dental Examiners, have naturally produced some modifications. Nonetheless, this public document stands alone as an excellent guidebook for dental managed care and will give the dentist-reader an important insight into how state regulatory agencies expect dental managed-care business to be handled, including the standards by which a managed-care provider should practice.

THE KNOX-KEENE DENTAL GUIDELINES
CALIFORNIA DEPARTMENT OF CORPORATIONS
HEALTH CARE SERVICE PLAN DIVISION:
SECTION 1, REGULATIONS

I. ACCESSIBILITY

Monitoring System

Each health-care service plan shall have a documented system for monitoring and evaluating accessibility of care, including a system for addressing problems that develop, which shall include but not be limited to, waiting time and appointments.

Information for Enrollees

A section of the health education program shall be designated to inform enrollees regarding accessibility of service in accordance with the needs of such enrollees for such information regarding that plan or area.

Communication

The plan shall provide translators and multilanguage directional signs and informational materials where more than 15% of the enrolled population receiving service at any one delivery site speaks a single language other than English.

Referrals

A plan shall provide accessibility to required dental specialists who are certified or eligible for certification by the appropriate specialty board, through staffing, contracting, or referral.

Written contracts must be executed between the plan and each provider of health-care services that regularly furnishes services under the plan.

Dental specialist care should be provided through direct contracting between the plan and specialist whenever possible. Referral arrangements through the general dentist (under capitation) may not adequately compensate the dentist to ensure proper referral of all cases requiring specialty care.

Staffing Patterns

Within each service area of a plan, the plan shall provide for the maintenance of staff, including health professionals, administrative and other supporting staff, directly or through an adequate referral system, sufficient to assure that health-care services will be provided on a timely and appropriate basis to enrollees.

There shall be at least one full-time equivalent dentist to each 2,000 enrollees, or an alternative mechanism shall be provided by the plan to demonstrate an adequate ratio of dentists to enrollees.

There shall be sufficient dental specialists (orthodontist, endodontist, periodontist, pediatric dentist, or oral surgeon) to allow patients to be referred and seen within two weeks.

Appointments

The plan shall encourage patients to be seen by appointment, except in emergencies.

A. Time-specific appointments for routine primary nonemergent care shall be available within two weeks.

B. Patients with more serious, acute, or urgent problems shall be triaged and provided same-day service if necessary or within 24 hours.

The plan has in effect an established policy that scheduled patients shall not routinely wait for more than 15–30 minutes to be seen by a provider.

Hours of operation and provision of after-hour services shall be reasonable, including emergency services.

The plan shall have an established policy and procedure for encouraging new enrollees to choose primary care dentists.

The location of facilities providing primary dental care services of the plan shall be within reasonable proximity of the business or personal residence of enrollees, and so located as not to result in unreasonable barriers to accessibility.

II. ACCEPTABILITY/ PUBLIC POLICY

Participation

In selection of enrollee and subscriber members of any governing board or standing committee, the plan shall consider makeup of its enrollee and subscriber population, including but not limited to, factors such as ethnic extraction, demography, occupation, and geography, as well as identifiable and individual group participation; any such selection or election of enrollee or subscriber members shall be conducted on a fair and reasonable basis.

These individuals who fulfill the requirements stated in this section for subscriber and/or enrollee membership upon the governing body or standing committee shall be persons who are not employees of the plan, providers of health-care services, subcontractors to the plan or group contract brokers, or persons financially interested in the plan.

Enrollees and subscribers participating in establishing public policy shall have access to information available from the plan regarding public policy, including financial information and information about the specific nature and volume of complaints received by the plan and their disposition.

The plan shall, at least annually, furnish to its subscribers and enrollees a description of its system for their participation in establishing public policy.

The plan shall communicate material changes affecting public policy to subscribers and enrollees.

Patient confidentiality shall be maintained in accordance with state and federal regulations.

The plan shall maintain confidentiality of patient records by defining who is to have access to records and for what purpose, obtaining written consent for release of medical/dental information, safeguarding against unauthorized use, and instructing plan employees in maintaining confidentiality.

III. CONTINUITY OF CARE

Referrals

Referrals shall include the timely sharing of all necessary information with health professionals to whom the patient is referred.

There shall be in effect an adequate system of documentation of referrals, including provision for timely and adequate information transfer to the plan and the responsibility for follow-up.

Broken Appointments Follow-up

The plan shall utilize a procedure for follow-up of broken appointments. This shall include a method for recognizing patterns of broken appointments so that action can be taken to alter those patterns.

IV. INTERNAL QUALITY OF CARE REVIEW SYSTEM

Peer Review

A plan shall conduct or cause to be conducted regular effective peer review that is practicable and reasonable, to identify and improve suboptimal professional performance with respect to diagnosis, treatment, quality and quantity of radiographs, and other aspects of the dental-care delivery process.

The plan shall assess the quality of dental care rendered by prospective providers prior to their enrollment as plan providers.

Dental Records

The professional staff shall conduct reviews for the adequacy and completeness of dental records.

Each dental plan shall maintain a dental record service with at least the following components:

- A numbering or other appropriate identifying system that uniquely identifies each patient

- A retrieval system through which an enrollee's dental record may be produced on demand

- A storage system that maintains inactive enrollee dental records in a specific place

- Dental records shall be legible to plan personnel and understandable; shall be organized; and all entries shall be dated and the responsible provider clearly identified

Quality of Care Audit

Plans shall have an operational quality of care review system to ensure quality health care by continually assessing and addressing problems, including care provided through primary care dentists and specialists.

The plan shall have a quality of care review system containing the attributes listed below:

- Identification of less than satisfactory performance of elements

Appendix I

of care, by considering information from all reasonably available sources, including, for example, peer review, dental record audits, enrollee assessment audits, grievances, and statistical reports

- Establishment of valid and achievable dental standards by health professional peers for those identified elements of dental care that are amenable to standard setting and compliance measurement

- Assurance that those standards that are established will be related to conditions that can be affected by dental care intervention, apply to a significant number of patients, and apply to all parts of the provider system, rather than just one class of providers

- Ratification, consensus, and documented communication of these topics, objectives, and criteria to all concerned

- Objective measurement of actual performance as reflected in data gathered from dental records, enrollee assessments, and other sources so as to include a representative sample of all such performance, in order to determine apparent noncompliance with standards

- Analysis by health professional peers of the results of objective measurement

- Implementation of necessary corrective action either immediate or routine, together with documentation thereof, and reports for additional dental, educational, or administrative action as appropriate

- Reaudit of actual performance after a specific scheduled interval to determine effectiveness of the remedial action, evaluation of the particular audit study documented, including problems identified, action taken, and results

- Periodic documented critical review of the design and ongoing implementation and effectiveness of the quality of care review system by the health professional peers and the plan's governing body

Utilization Review

The plan shall design and implement reasonable procedures for review of utilization of services and facilities, and costs.

V. FACILITY, PERSONNEL, AND EQUIPMENT LICENSURE

Personnel Licensure/Certification

All personnel employed by or under contract to the plan shall be licensed or certified by their respective board or agency where required by law.

Equipment Licensure

All equipment required to be licensed or registered by law shall be so licensed or registered and the operating personnel for such equipment shall be licensed or certified as required by law.

Deficiencies identified by licensing and accrediting boards or agencies shall be corrected.

Licensing

Deficiencies identified by licensing and accrediting boards or agencies shall be corrected.

Safety

The plan shall have a written plan for response to fire and other disasters and/or emergencies.

Allied Health Personnel

The plan shall employ and utilize allied health manpower for the furnishing of services to the extent permitted by law and consistent with good dental practice.

Radiology Safety

Where X-rays are taken on the premises, there is an established policy with regard to radiological safety, which includes:

- Periodic inspections of all X-ray shielding and equipment are made by a state or local radiological health authority as required by state law, and also when new equipment is installed or changes made in the structural design of the radiology department

- Identified hazards are promptly corrected

Sterilization and Disinfection

(This section of the guidelines has been superseded by current OSHA, Cal-OSHA, and CDC guidelines.)

Cleanliness

Offices shall be neat in appearance, be in good repair, and have pleasant and comfortable waiting areas.

Operatories shall be clean and neat in appearance, free from dust and dirt on the floors, on instrumentation, and on counters and drawers.

Cast rooms and other working areas shall be maintained in good repair, free from excessive debris, dust, and plaster.

Medical Emergency Preparedness

There shall be, on the premises, an emergency oxygen source with an operative pressure regulator and reservoir bag.

Emergency drug kits shall be maintained up to dately.

There shall be established procedures for obtaining outside medical emergency assistance.

Staff shall be trained in the administration of emergency oxygen and drugs; staff shall also be knowledgeable in procedures for obtaining outside emergency assistance.

Mercury Safety

Amalgam shall be prepared in amalgamators that prevent spillage and are not hazardous to one's health.

Mercury drops and amalgam scraps shall be immediately collected and properly stored in a tightly closed container and immersed in an appropriate solution.

VI. GRIEVANCE SYSTEM

Format/Records/Files

The plan shall have a formal subscriber/enrollee grievance procedure (format must be approved by the commissioner) to include steps for problem rectification when appropriate, and also procedures for the receipt, handling, and disposition of complaints whether said complaints were made at a grievance location, by letter, or by telephone. The grievance record shall include:

- Date of complaint
- Identification of the individual making the complaint
- Nature of the complaint
- Disposition of the complaint

The plan shall keep in its files copies of all complaints, and its responses thereto, for at least five years.

Notification of Subscribers and Enrollees

The plan shall inform its subscribers and enrollees on enrollment in the plan and annually thereafter of the procedure for processing and resolving grievances.

Grievance Process

Complaint forms and a copy of the grievance procedure shall be readily available at each plan facility (including facilities of providers) and furnished promptly on request, by mail or telephone.

Grievance Filing

Assistance shall be provided at each grievance location for filing grievances ("patient advocate" or "ombudsman" may be used).

Telephone Number/Grievance Location

The plan shall have one telephone number located in each service area (including major facilities that are extensively used by the plan) for the filing of complaints.

Primary Responsibility

An officer of the plan (designated in writing) shall have the primary responsibility to maintain grievance procedures, review the operations of the system, recognize and use emergent patterns of grievances in the formulation of policy changes and changes in plan procedures and operations.

There shall be prompt review of complaints by management or supervisory staff responsible for services or operations that are the subject of complaint.

Periodic Documentation of System

The review procedure of the grievance system, including documentation of the procedure or mechanism used in tabulating and reviewing patterns of grievances regularly, shall itself be carried out periodically and documented.

Discrimination

The plan shall assure that there is no discrimination against an enrollee or a subscriber (including cancellation of the contract) solely on the grounds that the enrollee filed a complaint.

Acknowledgment and Disposition

A grievance system shall provide: (a) for the acknowledgment to the receipt of a complaint and notice to the complainant who may be contacted with respect thereto within 20 days, and (b) for notice to complainant of disposition of the complaint normally within 30 days. Where the plan is unable to distinguish between complaints and inquiries, they shall be considered complaints.

THE KNOX-KEENE DENTAL GUIDELINES CALIFORNIA DEPARTMENT OF CORPORATIONS HEALTH CARE SERVICE PLAN DIVISION: SECTION 2, QUALITY OF CARE

HISTORY AND CLINICAL EXAMINATION

The dental history and clinical examination should focus on the problem or complaint presented by the patient. The dental history and clinical examination should also include a general survey of the oral cavity and related structures.

The dental history and clinical examination records, or charts, should include a tooth chart indicating the oral condition as to:

- Caries
- Restorations, defective or acceptable
- Fixed and removable prostheses
- Missing teeth
- Documentation on the status of missing, filled, and decayed teeth should be recorded at the first initial-care visit
- Endodontic status
- Documentation of soft tissue examination shall be done; documentation of positive or negative soft tissue findings, including oral cancer examination, shall be recorded at the first initial-care visit and at the first visit of maintenance care
- Periodontal status, based on minimal probing and screening; existing conditions including location and measurement of pockets, etiologic factors, mobile teeth, occlusal trauma
- Occlusal status
- Description of the general health and appearance of the neck, lips, gingiva, oral mucosal membranes, tongue, pharynx; evidence of attrition and erosion, bruxism or clenching, harmful habits; and attitude
- Incipient and other types of lesions

The medical history should allow for a thorough physical evaluation of the patient's physical and emotional ability to tolerate dental procedures safely, as well as a general evaluation of his health.

The general medical history should contain information pertaining to:

- General health and appearance
- Systemic diseases, such as cardiac condition, history of rheumatic fever, diabetes, hepatitis, venereal disease, and AIDS

Appendix I

- Allergies and sensitivity to drugs
- Reaction to dental anesthetics
- Present medication and present treatment
- Bleeding problems
- Nervous disorders
- Any other pertinent information

All questions on the history forms should be completed with an appropriate response. No questions should be left blank.

Written evidence of follow-up should be present for all patients with significant positive findings.

Medical alerts should appear on the outside of every patient folder when significant medical problems are present.

Based upon review of the medical history, and completion of the physical evaluation, the physical status of the patient may be graded in accord with the American Society of Anesthesiologists' classification:

Class 1: A normal healthy patient for an elective procedure

Class 2: A patient with mild systemic disease

Class 3: A patient with severe systemic disease that limits activity but is not incapacitating

Class 4: A patient with an incapacitating disease that is a constant threat to life

Class 5: A moribund patient who is not expected to survive for 24 hours

The medical and dental history should be updated periodically. Documentation of updated medical histories should occur with all patients at recall. Baseline observations should be recorded for comparison with future observations as the patient returns for periodic examination and treatment.

RADIOGRAPHS

- Initial full radiographic series for adults with dentition shall include 14 or more periapical films with necessary bitewing films, or a panographic film with bitewing films and periapical films, as necessary.

- A full radiographic series for edentulous adults, if a periapical series is not preferred, shall include occlusal films with molar-region periapical films, or a panographic film supplemented with all necessary periapical films in questioned regions.
- Initial radiographic series for children, prior to the eruption of the permanent second molars, shall include those periapical and bitewing films or a panographic film or lateral jaw film and those bitewing films that are necessary to depict the erupted and developing dentition, commensurate with the age of the patient.
- Recall and/or posttreatment radiographs are not to be taken on a routine basis, but rather, on an individual basis, depending on the individual's age, general or systemic condition, and his or her proneness to caries or periodontal change. Recall radiographs are justified in the presence of questioned pulpal or periapical responses, embedded or impacted teeth, questioned bone change, and delayed development of eruption of the dentition. In these instances, bitewing films or single periapical films of the questioned regions are to be used rather than full series.
- A full radiographic series should not be taken more than once every three years unless there are specific indications for more frequent examinations.
- A bitewing film series should not be taken more than once in a 12-month period unless there are specific indications for more frequent examinations.
- Radiographs should be kept on file for reference in subsequent evaluations and treatment and should be reviewed on a regular basis, considering not only proposed treatment, but also treatment performed in the past.
- For evaluation or treatment of specific sites, such as extraction of third molars, single films, panographic films, or lateral jaw films shall be used. Additional films shall not be taken with a

full intraoral periapical series unless there are specific indications for additional information unattainable with single intraoral films.

- Films must be taken in compliance with state and federal regulations for radiation hygiene.
- Original or duplicate films shall be forwarded on patient referral or transferred to another practitioner to prevent or minimize need for reexposure to radiation. The use of double film packets or photographic duplication is recommended for maintaining file records.
- In carefully selected cases in which a particular service is in question, postoperative radiographs may be required on an individual basis.

Radiographs shall be of such quality that:

- Standard illumination permits differentiation between the various structures of the teeth, the periodontal ligament spacings, the supporting bone, and normal anatomic landmarks.
- All crowns and roots, including apices, are fully depicted together with interproximal alveolar crests, contact areas, and surrounding bone regions.
- Images of all teeth and other structures are shown in proper relative size and contour with minimal distortion and without overlapping images where anatomically possible.

DIAGNOSIS

- Complete written diagnostic notations shall be made and symbolic tooth charting used to indicate pathological conditions.
- Consultations and referrals shall occur where necessary to complete diagnosis, with written reports on additional findings.
- The diagnosis shall be complete as evidenced and supported by recording major clinical symptoms and conditions.

TREATMENT PLANNING

Treatment plans should follow a logical sequence, such as:

- Relief of pain and discomfort
- Elimination of infection, irritations, traumatic conditions
- Treatment of extensive carious lesions and pulpal inflammation
- Prophylaxis and instruction in preventive practices
- Periodontal treatment
- Elimination of remaining caries and necessary extractions
- Restoration and replacement of teeth
- Placement of the patient on a recall schedule to suit the assessed needs
- Selection of antimicrobials shall be based on identification and sensitivity of the infecting organism as well as the efficacy of the agent and its potential adverse effects on the patient
- Final restoration of a tooth or teeth requiring endodontic and/or periodontal treatment should be postponed until a favorable prognosis for the retention of the tooth or teeth has been established
- The plan of treatment shall include an optimal amount of treatment at any single appointment and is based on the requirements for a functional dentition and a healthy oral cavity
- Outpatient management shall be planned unless, in the judgment of the dentist, the severity of the disease, complexity of the treatment, or health of the patient warrants hospitalization
- The plan of treatment should include consultation and/or referral for treatment when the nature of the disease, complexity of treatment, or health of the patient is beyond the normal scope of any particular dentist
- The dentist shall inform the patient of the diagnosis, recommended plan of treatment, prognosis, and complications

- The treatment plan and procedures shall be written systematically in the patient's record before treatment is started
- Where only operative procedures, such as restorations, are planned, symbolic charting will suffice as a treatment plan

PREVENTIVE DENTISTRY

Caries Prevention

- There shall be a comprehensive program of plaque control geared to the individual patient's susceptibility to caries.
- There shall be noted recommendations for the use of systemic fluoride, fluoride toothpaste, and/or fluoride rinse where indicated.
- There shall be noted recommendations of sealants and treatment plan including sealants where there is evidence of potential pit and fissure caries in an otherwise healthy, nonfilled tooth.

Periodontal Disease Prevention

- A comprehensive program of plaque removal and control shall be maintained along with other procedures, such as: prophylaxis, dental health education, occlusal evaluation, correcting malocclusions and malposed teeth, restoring broken down and deformed teeth, replacing missing teeth, and requiring the patient to practice thorough plaque control.
- There shall be evidence of plaque control instruction, evaluation, and follow-up.
- There shall be evidence of examination of periodontal pocket depths and bleeding and follow-up.
- No visible stains or bacterial plaque shall remain on the teeth following use of disclosing media.
- Supragingival and subgingival calculus shall be removed regardless of their location.

Prevention of Other Oral Diseases

Recognition of potentially harmful tissue changes shall be the responsibility of the dental practitioner. Prevention of systemic complications:

- Determining the physical and emotional ability of a particular patient to tolerate a specific dental procedure is the responsibility of the dentist.

ENDODONTICS

- Examination of the endodontic patient should include an evaluation of the pain and the stimuli that induce or relieve pain.

- Treatment planning shall include the strategic importance of the tooth or teeth considered for treatment, the prognosis, and such other factors as excessively curved canals, periodontal disease, occlusion, tooth fractures, and calcified or occluded canals. Teeth that are predisposed to fracture following endodontic treatment should be adequately protected.

Endodontic services may include vital pulp and root canal treatments.

Vital Pulp Treatment

- Indirect pulp capping may be indicated in the presence of deep carious lesions when there is evidence of vital and normal pulp tissue. Adequate radiographic evidence of protective reparative dentin formations shall be used to complete treatment.

- Direct pulp capping may be indicated in the presence of a small exposed vital or normal pulp.

- Pulpotomy may be indicated in permanent teeth when there is evidence of a vital and normal pulp in order to maintain pulp vitality in the immature permanent root or roots and promote maturation of the root. When the root is fully formed, endodontic treatment shall be completed.

- Pulpotomy may be indicated on deciduous teeth when there is a reasonable residual period of retention and function of the deciduous tooth and when the pulp pathosis is confined to the coronal portion or when there is a pulp exposure too large for capping.
- Pulpectomy
- Nonsurgical treatment of root canals and pulp chambers
- Surgical treatment of periapical and lateral pathosis of pulpal origin
- Apicoectomy
- Replantation of teeth
- Endodontic implants

Factors which shall be considered in determining the acceptability of vital pulp treatment are:

- Radiographic evidence of calcification, i.e., reparative dentin formation for pulp capping and root apex maturation for pulpotomy
- The absence of tooth supportive structure changes
- A normal vital pulp response for pulp capping

Root Canal Treatment

Root canal treatment may be indicated on teeth with diseased or potentially diseased pulp with or without evidence of periapical pathosis. Treatment procedures consist of:

- Acceptable access
- Biomechanical cleansing and the shaping of the canal system
- Culturing when indicated
- Obturation of pulp chamber and canal system with suitable radiopaque material

These procedures should be performed under rubber dam isolation whenever feasible.

Nonsurgical Root Canal Treatment

- Apexification treatment may be indicated on a tooth with a necrotic pulp that has an immature root. The treatment involves the induction of apical closure over a period of several months. When closure is complete, normal endodontic therapy is performed.

Surgical Root Canal Treatment

Surgical treatment may be indicated when:

- The root canal system cannot be acceptably treated nonsurgically
- There is active root resorption
- Access to the root is obstructed
- There is gross overextension or underextension of the root canal filling
- Periapical or lateral pathosis persists
- There is a fracture of the root
- There is periodontal involvement requiring root amputation or hemisection
- Hemisection may be indicated when there is a fracture dividing the crown and/or roots or there is extensive loss of bone support for one or more of the roots and retention of one-half of the tooth is considered necessary for maintenance of function.
- Root amputation may be indicated on multirooted teeth when there is extensive loss of bone support on one root and amputation will significantly aid the periodontal condition and the patient's access for cleaning the involved area. Root canal treatment on the retained portions of the canal system is preferably completed prior to hemisection or root amputation.
- Replantation of a tooth may be indicated when the canal system is not accessible and owing to anatomic considerations apical surgery in situ is not advisable. Teeth that have been accidentally avulsed from the alveolus may be replanted to their original

position. Root canal treatment is performed prior to or after replantation.

Occlusal adjustment and stabilization may be necessary. All replanted teeth may show varying signs of root resorption. Failure of the replanted tooth from root resorption may occur in two or more years. The degree or extent of root resorption increases the longer the time interval for returning the tooth to its alveolus.

Treatment should result in the following:

- Tooth or teeth shall be asymptomatic
- There is evidence of reparative dentin formation
- Vital pulp response
- The endodontic filling is dense and obliterates the canal system
- Tooth or teeth treated are functional and nonmobile

PERIODONTICS

Periodontics consists of the diagnosis, treatment, and prevention of pathologic conditions affecting the supporting tissues of the teeth, including the gingiva, the periodontal ligament, and the alveolar bone.

The clinical examination of the periodontal patient should record the presence or absence of inflammatory and noninflammatory abnormalities, the condition and stability of the dentition, and the depth of the periodontal pockets.

Radiographs are used to evaluate the condition and amount of alveolar bone in conjunction with manual probing and measurements of pockets.

Children and adolescents should be screened for evidence of periodontal disease. Adult patients should be examined, probed, and charted to provide baseline information of the periodontal condition and informed of the presence of any periodontal disease.

A notation shall be made in the patient's record as to whether or not the dentist treats the condition, refers the patient, or the patient does not elect treatment at the time. Existing conditions shall be recorded and should include:

- Location and measurement of pockets

- Etiologic factors
- Mobile teeth
- Occlusal trauma

Root planing and scaling should result in:

- Removal of irregularities, roughness, and deposits
- Smoothing of roots

Periodontal surgery may be accomplished by a variety of procedures. In gingival curettage, the following services should be accomplished under anesthesia:

- Removal of soft tissue comprising the sulcular wall along with any residual calculus, granulation tissue, or debris when indicated
- Correction of inflammation as evidenced by bleeding or purulence upon probing
- Gingivectomy, flap, osseous, mucogingival, and all other periodontal surgery should result in the elimination of periodontal pathosis. The gingiva should be restored to appropriate physiologic form commensurate with health.

Deformities in the alveolar bone are corrected by:

- Reshaping
- Grafts or curettage of the bony defects that would tend to regenerate bone for repair

Following treatment, clinical examination should evidence:

- Healthy tissues
- Absence of inflammation
- Acceptable gingival form
- Absence of bacterial plaque or calculus
- A nontraumatic occlusion

The patient should be treated in skills for plaque-control procedures. A follow-up program for evaluation of the success of treatment,

Appendix I

continuous supportive therapy, and maintenance program should be established.

- Patients should be recalled for periodic prophylaxis and periodontal evaluation depending on their individual rate of plaque and calculus formation.
- The condition of the periodontal tissues, the depth of pockets, and the course of treatment should be recorded on appropriate charts periodically.

ORAL AND MAXILLOFACIAL SURGERY

Preventive Measures

- There shall be provisions for management of medical, surgical, or dental emergencies.
- There shall be acceptable methods of prophylaxis utilized to prevent medical complications.
- There shall be standards of asepsis including autoclaving of all surgical instruments, utilization of single-use injection needles, cleanliness of treatment areas, and aseptic scrub and surgical techniques, which include sterile gloves and drapes and surgical scrub of the hands and operative sites.
- All tissues removed at surgery shall be identified macroscopically and/or microscopically. Immediate definitive care is mandated by suspected malignancy or other life-threatening conditions.
- There shall be removal of malpositioned and impacted teeth that are regarded as pathologic by virtue of their position. Corrective surgical intervention may be indicated as determined by clinical and radiographic examination by the treating dentist with the following exceptions:
    - Teeth with potential for replacement of diseased or compromised adjacent teeth

- Teeth that can be brought into position orthodontically, when that modality is indicated and planned
- Those unusual conditions where the health interests of the patient are served by retention of the teeth in question

There shall be provision for scheduled follow-up and observation.

Therapeutic Measures

- Dental extractions are based on a clearly recorded diagnosis for which extraction is treatment choice of the dentist and patient. Extractions may be indicated in the presence of nonrestorable caries, untreatable periodontal disease, pulpal and periapical disease not amenable to endodontic therapy, and malposed, unerupted, or impacted teeth, or when overriding medical conditions exist that provide compelling justification to eliminate existing or potential sources of oral infection.

- Tissue management includes flap design appropriate to the surgical procedure, bone removal accomplished with acceptable surgical methods, tooth sectioning when indicated, reapproximation of displaced tissue to avoid exposed bone, and use of pressure dressings and other supportive measures when indicated.

- Completion of the procedure includes all portions of extracted teeth having been removed unless contraindicated, contouring of bone supporting soft tissue to reduce postoperative sequelae, recording of unanticipated sequelae such as failure to remove planned tissue or organs, unplanned removal of tissue or organs, displacement of tissue or organs to abnormal sites, unusual blood loss, etc., absence of lacerations, and other surgical or nonsurgical defects.

Supportive Care

- Management of the oral surgery patient requires many adjunctive elements related to the surgical treatment.

- Nonsurgical treatment of temporomandibular joint abnormalities directed toward elimination of etiologic factors as well as

alleviation of symptoms whether in support of surgical treatment or as the primary means of treatment.
- Appliances for the immobilization of oral structures to provide good stabilization of the intended parts, whether in treatment of traumatic injury, as adjunctive care in oncologic surgery, or other conditions requiring such appliances (minimal injury to the tissues is caused by the appliances).

There shall be:

- Provisions for postoperative care and for treatment of complications
- Written reports to referring practitioner for patients seen on consultation
- Written directions for home care in the treatment not requiring active therapy

Crowns and Fixed Partial Prosthodontics

- Crowns include the following acceptable restorations: full crowns, seven-eighths crowns, three-quarters crowns, and onlays. Also included are porcelain and plastic crowns used as a single material or in combination with acceptable cast metal.
- A thorough history and clinical examination leading to the diagnosis of the patient's general and oral condition must be completed before establishing a treatment plan. Care must be exercised when placing crowns so that the hardness of the material used is compatible with that of the opposing dentition.

A conservative treatment plan shall be considered prior to providing the patient with one or more crowns. Amalgam or composite restorations may be inappropriate for the following reasons:

- The restoration will receive excessive masticatory force that might fracture the remaining tooth structure or restorations
- There is a fractured or missing cusp or incisal edge
- Seventy-five percent of the tooth surface is a series of restorations

(amalgam, silicate, or composite), one or more of which is defective, or an additional carious lesion is present

- There is gross decay on all tooth surfaces
- Tooth with completed root canal therapy that cannot be restored and maintained with amalgam, silicate, or composite materials
- Patient has a significant loss of vertical dimension of tooth structure with heavily abraded occlusal surfaces, and corrective equilibration will not stop further loss of tooth structure
- Patient has a failing crown that can only be restored by another crown
- The teeth are to be splinted

A final restoration of a tooth or teeth that requires endodontic and/or periodontic treatment should be postponed until a favorable prognosis for the retention of the tooth or teeth has been established.

Crown(s) must be incorporated in the treatment plan in the appropriate sequence in relation to endodontic, periodontic, and surgical procedures. When serious unsightly tooth appearance exists, porcelain or plastic jacket crowns (often combined with metal) may be used to improve aesthetics and are acceptable restorations when aesthetics are the primary concern.

Restorations should exhibit contours that are in functional harmony with adjacent teeth and soft tissues, exhibiting good individual anatomic form, with no food traps or soft tissue irritation present, and design should facilitate good oral hygiene.

Fixed partial prostheses are indicated for replacement of one or more missing teeth when abutment teeth can be expected to have a minimum prognosis of five years of service.

Cast crowns and porcelain jacket crowns as well as fixed partial prostheses are contraindicated when:

- The necessary operative procedures impair the patient's oral health
- The necessary operative procedures inhibit growth and development
- There is no clear rationale for improving or stabilizing present dental function

Appendix I

- The patient is under 16 years of age, unless unusual conditions prevail
- Second and third molars, with rare exceptions, are not replaced unless they are part of a bridge restoring other missing teeth
- There shall be no discoloration on the margin between the restoration and tooth surface
- Restoration satisfies operative dentistry principles of margin placement wherever possible
- There shall be no visible evidence of a crevice along the margin into which an explorer will penetrate

REMOVABLE PARTIAL PROSTHODONTICS

- Removable partial prosthodontics is that part of dental practice that deals with the restoration of the occlusion by means of removable appliances, which may be either entirely tooth supported or tooth and tissue supported. The appliance generally derives its support principally from tissues underlying its base with a lesser amount of support from some remaining teeth.
- Removable partials are indicated when the initial history, clinical examination, and diagnosis reveal conditions that contraindicate replacement of missing teeth with fixed prosthetic appliances or when individual patient factors preclude fixed prosthetic restorations.
- A removable partial denture is normally not indicated for a single tooth replacement as a permanent restoration or as a replacement of nonfunctional second and third molars.

Properly constructed fixed restorations are usually more physiologically and psychologically acceptable to the patient. Conditions that may contraindicate fixed restorations are:

- Replacement of two or more teeth when distal abutment tooth is missing

- Replacement of missing teeth in cases of periodontal involvement of remaining teeth with unfavorable prognosis
- Replacement of an anterior tooth or teeth immediately following extraction when a temporary plastic appliance will provide adequate aesthetics during the healing period
- Use as a provisional appliance where final diagnosis cannot be made
- Replacement of missing anterior teeth where aesthetics are better served by a removable partial denture
- Where edentulous areas are too extensive and/or resorbed to be successfully restored by fixed partial prostheses

Materials used for removable partial prostheses must be strong enough to resist bending or breakage during normal function, nonporous, color stable, aesthetically pleasing, nontoxic, and nonabrading to the supporting dentition.

Design shall provide for satisfactory saddle-area coverage, functional stability, noninterfering functional occlusion, and passive retention when not in function. Consideration should always be given to bilateral support of removable partial prostheses. Appliances are designed to cause no damage to abutment teeth and/or periodontal tissues, and to facilitate oral hygiene.

The prostheses shall function passively, fit the natural teeth accurately, be well adapted to the soft tissues, and provide increased masticatory function for the patient.

COMPLETE DENTURE PROSTHODONTICS

Complete dentures are the restoration of last resort. They are indicated as a treatment procedure only when the prognosis for the remaining teeth is hopeless, or when all upper or lower teeth have been removed.

Complete dentures are important not only for improved mastication of food, but also for proper facial appearance and speech. The construction of complete dentures is as much an art as it is a science. The psychological management of the patient may be of greater importance

Appendix I

than the technical aspects of the complete denture service. Technically acceptable dentures may be a complete failure because the psychological limitations of the patient were not recognized. In situations where findings do not meet satisfactory criteria but where a patient is completely satisfied with function and appearance and no pathology is present, the denture is considered to be satisfactory.

Severely handicapped edentulous patients, either physically or emotionally or both, may require special procedures based upon the problems they present. Patients should be referred for treatment of conditions beyond the skills of the treating dentist.

Aesthetically, the denture should harmonize with the patient's facial appearance. Position, size, and shade of teeth appear natural and unobtrusive. The color and the shade of the denture base material should appear natural and unobtrusive.

Complete dentures should exhibit proper peripheral seal at the mucobuccal fold and cover those areas of the arches that provide maximum support.

The maxillary denture should cover the hard palate, with a postdam that extends from the hamular notch to form a posterior seal on the soft palate without evidence of inflammation or ulceration.

The mandibular denture should have full posterior flanges, normally extending to or beyond the floor of the mouth and extending distally to include a portion or all of the retromolar pad.

The denture base material should adapt closely to the soft tissues and extension should achieve stability without evidence of inflammation or ulceration.

Centric occlusion should be in harmony with centric jaw relation in the most closed position of the teeth. Vertical dimension of occlusion should be within the physiologic tolerance of the patient. Interocclusal contacts should be evenly distributed with no occlusal interference in lateral or protrusive excursions. The dentures should remain seated when biting pressure is applied in the anterior and posterior segments of the arch and during talking and smiling.

Postinsertion care may involve adjustment of the denture base or the occlusion, or resetting or changing teeth. It may also involve relining of the denture if there is inadequate adaption of the denture base to the tissues. The treatment plan should include provision for postinsertion care with the dentist accepting responsibility for rendering this care for a period of six months. Porcelain or plastic are acceptable materials for artificial teeth. In selected cases, metal occlusal surfaces may be indicated. The use of plastic teeth opposing cast restorations is recommended.

The same guidelines should apply to immediate complete dentures as to remote complete dentures. One exception is the indication in some immediate denture cases for reduction or eliminating the labial flange of the denture. The dentist has the responsibility of informing the patient of the necessity for modifying the denture at periodic intervals to compensate for the tissue changes that will occur.

PEDODONTICS

Pedodontics is that part of dental practice that deals with the growth and development of the dentition and the diagnosis and treatment of dental disease in children and adolescents.

There should be particular concern to preserve the primary teeth for masticatory function and space maintenance, utilizing such procedures as pulpal therapy and stainless steel crowns.

To preserve adequate space for the eruption of the permanent dentition, both space maintainers and space regainers should be employed judiciously, with particular preference for fixed appliances.

Tooth guidance and regulation of the growth and development of the dentition is also an important feature of pedodontic care. Patients should be referred for treatment of conditions beyond the skill of the treating dentist.

Excessive and unnecessary treatment should be avoided. For example, carious lesions of primary incisors that will exfoliate within six to nine months should not be restored unless it is warranted by special circumstances. Routine administration of premedications should be avoided for tractable children. Inhalation sedation and/or premedication may be used selectively when indicated for management of pain and anxiety.

Principles and practices of prevention should be employed, such as dietary counseling and plaque control. Topical fluorides should be applied at least annually as part of the prophylaxis, and dietary fluorides should be prescribed where the water supplies are deficient. Application of sealants should be utilized where appropriate.

Appendix I

ORTHODONTICS

- Orthodontics includes space maintenance, tooth guidance, interceptive procedures, and full orthodontic treatment to influence growth with orthopedic forces as well as to influence the positions of individual teeth. Removable and/or fixed appliances may be used to accomplish these goals. Candidates for orthodontic treatment should be in good oral health.

- Of particular importance is the timing of treatment, which may be initiated in the deciduous dentition, the mixed dentition, or the adult dentition. Orthodontics may be completed in one or more phases of treatment.

- The principles and practices of prevention should be employed in the diagnosis and treatment of orthodontic problems, including informing the patient of the advisability of dietary counseling and plaque control, and the application of topical fluorides prior to the placement of orthodontic appliances and at appropriate intervals thereafter.

- The final results of orthodontic treatment should be directed towards the attainment of an optimal end-result for each patient with regard to dentition, supporting bone relationship, interdigitation, contact points, overbite, and overjet to achieve aesthetic improvement and stability of attained correction. Active orthodontic treatment should be followed with retention appliances and supervision to help assure stability of correction.

- A satisfactory result in orthodontics is dependent upon the combination of professional skill and patient cooperation during all phases of treatment, considering the age of the patient, the severity of the presenting malocclusion, the desired treatment objectives, as well as individual osteogenic patterns during treatment.

- Baseline conditions shall be recorded by means of radiographs (including at least one cephalogram and its analysis), study casts oriented in centric relation, intraoral and extraoral photographs, a complete oral examination, and a complete dental, medical, and family history. Oral myological or myofunctional evaluation should be performed as necessary.

- The appliances and treatments used shall be appropriate for the treatment of the orthodontic problems.
- Appliances fit well. Bands are adapted and cemented so that cement margins are barely visible.
- The end results for treatment meet accepted norms for function and exhibit a balanced and stable skeletal, facial, and dental arch form optimal for the patient.
- Axial inclination of the anterior and posterior teeth are such that optimal aesthetic and functional results are achieved.
- Interproximal spaces (contacts) are closed.
- There is no significant gingival recession, evidence of loss of supporting bone, root resorption, caries, or decalcification of the teeth.

Appendix II

A Sample Dental Provider Agreement

This Contract dated this _____ day of _____, 19 _____, by and between _____ (hereinafter referred to as "DENTIST") and ABC Dental Plan, Inc. (hereinafter referred to as "ABC") is made with reference to the following facts:

  A. ABC provides various groups and organizations with dental care for their members and dependents, as defined herein. Said services are provided on a prepaid closed panel basis.

  B. Each of the groups represented by ABC has entered into a Benefit Agreement with ABC by the terms of which ABC has agreed to provide members and dependents, as defined herein, of each group with dental care and services as set forth in the particular Benefit Agreement, in exchange for periodic prepayment fees.

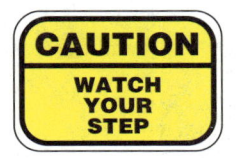

CAUTION WATCH YOUR STEP

Review the discussion on benefit agreements!

173

C. It is specifically understood by the parties hereto that the Benefit Agreements referred to in paragraph B above contain provisions which may vary in each Benefit Agreement and that said Benefit Agreements may be modified prospectively from time to time.

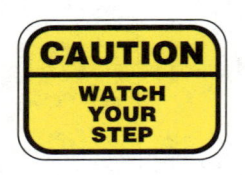

CAUTION WATCH YOUR STEP

Can the provider renegotiate the agreement accordingly?

D. It is further understood that ABC may enter into new Benefit Agreements with new groups during the term of this Contract and that DENTIST may be responsible for the provision of dental services under these new Benefit Agreements as provided herein, subject to the terms and conditions set forth in this Contract.

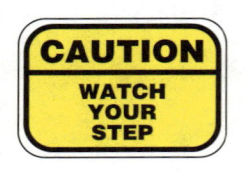

CAUTION WATCH YOUR STEP

These "new" benefit agreements can add up!

E. Neither ABC nor DENTIST shall discriminate against any provider or patient on the basis of race, national origin, sex, sexual orientation, physical handicap, or age.

NOW, THEREFORE, the parties do mutually covenant and agree as follows:

PART 1. DEFINITIONS

"Benefit Agreement" means the written agreement entered into between ABC and groups, under which ABC provides, indemnifies, or administers dental benefits to persons or groups.

"Capitation" means a uniform prepayment fee due the DENTIST, per Member, per month, based on the Benefit Agreement issued to the Member and the services available to the Member pursuant to this Benefit Agreement.

Appendix II

"Contract" means this agreement between DENTIST and ABC.

"Co-payment" means the additional charges due from the Member for Covered Dental Services.

"Covered Dental Services" means the services and benefits covered under the Benefit Agreement.

"Dental Director" means a licensed Dentist who is contracted or employed by ABC to provide professional advice concerning the operation of the Benefit Agreements.

"Dentist" means an individual who is licensed as a Doctor of Dental Surgery (D.D.S.) or Doctor of Dental Medicine (D.M.D.) in accordance with applicable state laws and who is practicing within the scope of such license, including any hygienists and technicians recognized by the dental profession who act and assist the Dentist.

"Dependent" shall mean the spouse and children, if enrolled in ABC, of a Member and shall include all newborn infants whose coverage shall commence from and after the moment of birth. Children are also subject to the applicable age limitations as established by each group or organization and any additional requirements in accordance with the Group Subscriber Agreement.

"Emergency" means a condition in which, in the opinion of the DENTIST, the Member has severe pain or symptoms which, if not treated immediately, would lead to unnecessary suffering, disability, or death.

"Emergency Services" means those Covered Dental Services provided in connection with an emergency.

"Exception" means any variance with the provisions of this Contract.

"Member" shall mean a person who is actually enrolled in ABC and eligible to receive services as provided for herein under a Benefit Agreement with ABC. The term "Member" or "Members" as used in this Contract shall be deemed to include all eligible Dependents of a Member as defined herein, if so enrolled in a Benefit Agreement with ABC.

"Peer Review Committee" means regional committees composed of

Dentists pursuant to the requirements of the Health Care Quality Improvement Act of 1986.

"Principal Benefits and Coverage with Co-payments" means those Covered Dental Services for which the Member has a co-payment.

"Principal Benefits and Coverage without Co-payments" means those Covered Dental Services for which the Member has no co-payment.

"Principal Excluded Procedures and Services" means those services which are specifically not Covered Dental Services.

"Principal Limitations" means those Covered Dental Services which are limited in frequency, number, or scope of treatment.

"Public Policy Committee" means an advisory committee composed of Dentists, Members, and members of ABC's Board of Directors.

"Special Notice" means communications requiring time deadline compliance by either party to this Contract sent by Certified Mail, Return Receipt Requested.

"Specialty Referral Guidelines" means specific procedures to be followed for Covered Dental Services provided by Dentists other than the DENTIST.

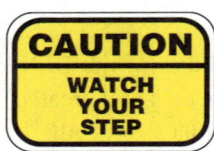

> ⚠ CAUTION — WATCH YOUR STEP: Get these guidelines placed in contract or incorporated by reference!

PART 2. RENDITION OF CARE

2.1   DENTIST agrees to promptly provide or arrange for all Covered Dental Services for each Member who has selected the DENTIST, in accordance with that Member's Benefit Agree-

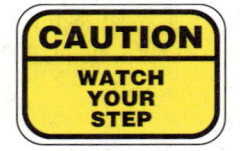

> ⚠ CAUTION — WATCH YOUR STEP: Each of these elements could be different in each benefit agreement!

Appendix II

ment, and to assure that those services are available and accessible in and through the facility of the DENTIST. The DENTIST shall have the right within the framework of professional ethics to reject any patient seeking his professional services. DENTIST agrees to expressly abide by the Principal Benefits and Coverage without Co-payments, Principal Benefits and Coverage with Co-payments, Principal Excluded Procedures and Services, and Principal Limitations contained within the said various Benefit Agreements.

2.2 It is agreed that DENTIST shall provide services during normal working hours and in addition, DENTIST agrees to provide Saturday hours and evening hours as may be necessary in order to keep patient appointment schedules on a reasonable, current basis.

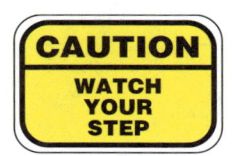

CAUTION — WATCH YOUR STEP

Determine your patient capacity first, or risk losing your weekends!

DENTIST shall also provide a 24-hour, seven days-a-week Emergency Service. ABC and DENTIST will mutually determine evening and Saturday hours in order to accomplish reasonable service in accordance with ABC's Benefit Agreement with the group. DENTIST also agrees that the office will be covered for Emergency Services during vacations and other periods when the office might be normally open.

2.3 DENTIST shall offer appointments to all Members upon request within a reasonable time. In nonemergency cases, a reasonable time shall not be more than two (2) weeks. In Emergency Cases, a reasonable time shall not be more than one day. In the event an individual is unable to obtain an appointment within a reasonable time, then after ABC has contacted the DENTIST, but is unable to mutually satisfy all parties concerned, then ABC shall be entitled to take whatever action is appropriate to obtain service within a reasonable time for the Member, and DENTIST shall be responsible for the costs or charges incurred for same.

2.4 ABC recognizes the Exception that circumstances may arise, beyond DENTIST'S control, which may make compliance with this provision impossible or impractical for a particular patient or for a limited period. The Dental Director shall approve or disapprove of this Exception.

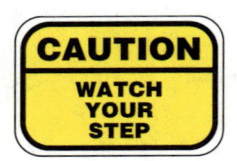

CAUTION — WATCH YOUR STEP

Is the dental director's decision final? Make sure appeals are present.

PART 3. ELIGIBILITY

3.1 All determinations as to the eligibility of any person, Member, or Dependent to receive Covered Dental Benefits under this Contract, or the standing of any person with respect to membership in any group or organization entitled to Covered Dental Benefits, shall be determined by the group and ABC before DENTIST renders any Covered Dental Benefits. ABC shall notify DENTIST whether such person is eligible for Covered Dental Benefits, and the nature and extent of Covered Dental Benefits to which such individual is entitled under his/her Benefit Agreement with the group.

3.2 ABC shall not be liable to DENTIST for any services rendered to persons not certified for services as herein provided. DENTIST shall follow ABC's procedures for determining which persons are eligible for services.

3.3 ABC shall provide DENTIST with an eligibility list updated monthly from which it can be determined who is eligible for services. In the event a Member claims to be eligible to receive Covered Dental Benefits, but whose name is not on the eligibility list forwarded by ABC to DENTIST, DENTIST shall contact ABC by telephone to ascertain whether said Member is eligible before refusing service to said Member.

Appendix II

ABC will guarantee eligibility in the event that the DENTIST is unable to reach ABC by telephone in an emergency situation.

Part 4. Services Not Covered; Fees Due Directly from Member

4.1 It is specifically understood and agreed that instances will arise where DENTIST will perform dental services which are either not covered by the Benefit Agreement then in force between the group and ABC (Principal Excluded Procedures and Services); for services for which the Benefit Agreement requires the Member to pay in whole or in part directly to the DENTIST (Principal Benefits and Coverage with Co-payments).

In such cases, Dentist agrees to look solely to the Member for payment for such services, and payment for such services shall be billed by DENTIST directly to the Member at a rate not to exceed the amount set forth in the Member's applicable schedules attached (Principal Benefits and Coverage with Co-payments), less any amount paid by group or such other insurance or other benefits covering said patient. **If additional services are required which are not listed in the "Principal Benefits and Coverage with Co-payments" and not listed as an excluded service, then the DENTIST agrees that the service is a covered benefit and no additional co-payment is required.** If the DENTIST'S charges for any services are estimated to exceed $250 per Member, then the DENTIST agrees to obtain a signed treatment agreement from the Member prior to the provision of those services.

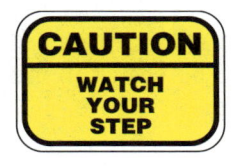

> **CAUTION — WATCH YOUR STEP**
>
> Never allow "covered benefits" to be determined by default, as shown here. They must be explicitly defined!

PART 5. BASIS OF PAYMENT TO DENTIST

5.1 ABC shall pay to DENTIST a monthly capitation payment which shall be payment for all services provided by DENTIST to Members of participating groups, other than those services for which charges are collected directly by DENTIST from Members as provided in Part 4.1 above. Such compensation shall be paid and mailed to the DENTIST on or before the 20th day of each month for services rendered during that month. Payment shall be based upon the number of Members of each group who selected the DENTIST'S facility, multiplied by the capitation rates for each applicable plan. The payment equals the total sum of each of the individual or group capitations.

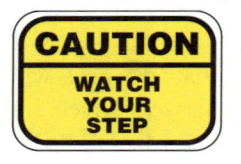

> **CAUTION — WATCH YOUR STEP**
>
> Be a good negotiator here. ABC wants to wait 20 days before paying you for services already rendered! Every day that you can accelerate payments is in your best interest!

5.2 DENTIST agrees that he/she will make no charge to the patient other than provided for in Part 4.1 above, and will look exclusively to ABC for periodic capitation payments.

5.3 COORDINATION OF BENEFITS: DENTIST shall comply with Exhibit A, which is attached hereto and made a part of this Contract.

PART 6. SPECIALIST; SUBSTITUTES

6.1 SUBSTITUTE DENTIST: Whenever DENTIST is on vacation or is to be absent for any extended period, DENTIST shall provide a substitute licensed dentist who shall be

Appendix II

responsible for the care and treatment of Members assigned to DENTIST. DENTIST shall be responsible for the capitation payment to such substitute dentist for services rendered to any eligible Member covered hereunder. In the event DENTIST fails to make necessary arrangements as provided for in this Part (6.1), ABC shall be entitled to take whatever action is appropriate to obtain services for the eligible person and DENTIST shall be responsible for the costs and charges incurred for same.

6.2 SPECIALIST REFERRALS: DENTIST agrees to abide by ABC's Specialty Referral Guidelines prior to initiating any referral requests.

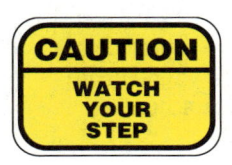

CAUTION — WATCH YOUR STEP

Remember to get all "guidelines" spelled out ...

  6.2-1 DENTIST agrees that in areas where ABC has arrangements in effect with a particular specialist or group of specialists, DENTIST shall refer eligible patients to such specialists for treatment. Failure to comply with this requirement may result in DENTIST assuming some portion of the treatment costs.

  6.2-2 DENTIST shall not be responsible for the charges incurred by a Member for any excluded services or procedures.

6.3 ORTHODONTIC REFERRALS: In the event a Member is in need of orthodontic services and orthodontic treatment is a Covered Dental Service under the Member's Benefit Agreement, DENTIST shall refer said Member to ABC who will arrange for treatment. DENTIST shall not be responsible for any charges incurred as a result of said orthodontic treatment, except for any treatment or services which otherwise would be a covered benefit under the Member's Benefit Agreement.

Part 7. Changes in Terms and Benefits Offered Groups

7.1   It is specifically understood that the benefits, terms, and conditions of the various Benefit Agreements between the participating groups and ABC may be changed from time to time during the term of this Contract. It is further understood that ABC may enter into Benefit Agreements with new groups or organizations during the term of this Contract for which the DENTIST will provide services to eligible persons as provided herein.

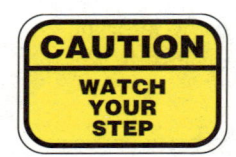

CAUTION WATCH YOUR STEP

Fine—but you and your attorney must be able to examine them and adjust the provider agreement accordingly!

Part 8. Term of Contract

8.1   This Contract will commence on the date set forth on page one of this Contract and shall be effective for a period of three (3) years from that date.

8.2   Following the initial three years of this Contract, the Contract shall automatically be renewed thereafter in additional three-year-term increments unless terminated sooner as provided in Part 16.

Part 9. Standard of Dental Care

9.1   DENTIST agrees that he/she shall perform all obligations under this Contract in accordance with high standards of

Appendix II

> **CAUTION**
> **WATCH YOUR STEP**

competence, care, and concern for the welfare and needs of the Members of the participating groups and in accordance with professional ethics, applicable state laws, and all other applicable state and federal regulations. In addition, the Standard of Care used to judge compliance with this section is the published guidelines of the state dental association, American Dental Association, and any additional written guidelines or standards developed by ABC's quality assurance committee or ABC's Dental Director. It is the responsibility of the DENTIST to obtain and maintain the current written Standards of Care for the State and region where the DENTIST's practice is located.

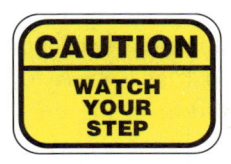

> **Get provision whereby you receive updates and changes to all applicable guidelines in Section 9.1**

9.2   DENTIST shall in no way differentiate the days and time of day when rendering professional care to Members of ABC and that of DENTIST's private patients.

9.3   It is understood that the inclusion of DENTIST on the panel of professional providers of each group or organization is not a recommendation of DENTIST by the group or organization, or of ABC.

Part 10. Nonexclusive Contract

10.1   This Contract is not exclusive in any respect. ABC, each participating group, and Members of such groups are entitled to enter into similar Contracts with other Dentists. DENTIST is also free to enter into agreements with other parties or with other groups not under Benefit Agreement with ABC and to conduct and maintain his/her private practice.

Part 11. Dentist/Patient Relationship

11.1   It is expressly understood that the relationship between the individual patients and DENTIST shall be subject to the rules, limitations, and privileges incident to the doctor/patient relationship.

11.2   DENTIST shall be solely responsible without interference from ABC or its agents to the Member for dental advice or treatment.

11.3   DENTIST shall have the right to refuse to treat any Member who violates the doctor/patient relationship. DENTIST must notify ABC immediately (Special Notice—Part 17) of the intention to invoke procedures of this Part 11.3; to refuse future service to any Member shall constitute a waiver of future capitation payments on behalf of the Member.

11.4   It is understood and agreed that the operation and maintenance of the dental offices, facilities and equipment, and the rendition of all dental services shall be solely and exclusively under the control and supervision of DENTIST. ABC shall have no right, authority, or control over either the selection of DENTIST'S staff, supervision of the personnel, the operation of the dental practice, or the rendition of any of the dental services. It is understood and agreed that nothing contained in this Contract shall be construed as giving ABC any right to manage or conduct the dental practice of DENTIST as a manager, proprietor, conductor, lessor, or otherwise.

11.5   DENTIST shall be solely responsible for all dental advice and services performed or prescribed for the Members. Neither ABC, its officers, directors, employees, administrators, agents, or representatives of ABC shall be liable for an act or omission of DENTIST or any agents, employees, or other persons performing services for or at the request of DENTIST.

Appendix II

11.6 There is not an employee/employer relationship between ABC and DENTIST. DENTIST shall provide dental services for ABC acting at all times as an independent contractor. ABC shall not be responsible to DENTIST or DENTIST'S employees, agents, or other persons performing services for or at the request of DENTIST for any salaries, payroll taxes, Worker's Compensation Insurance benefits or any other benefits.

11.7 Disagreements between the DENTIST and any Member regarding the Member's Benefit Agreement and/or the Covered Dental Services shall be resolved by requesting an opinion from the Dental Director, subject to the decisions of ABC's Peer Review Committee and Public Policy Committees regarding the Standard of Care and the scope of the Covered Dental Services. Both the DENTIST and the Member may appeal the decision of the Dental Director by making such an appeal within thirty (30) days in writing following the directions in Part 17 (Special Notices) to ABC's Peer Review Committee.

PART 12. PROFESSIONAL LIABILITY INSURANCE; IMMUNITY FROM LIABILITY

12.1 INSURANCE: DENTIST agrees to maintain in full force and effect during the term of the Contract, general liability insurance and professional liability insurance in an amount not less than Two Hundred Thousand Dollars ($200,000) per incident and/or Five Hundred Thousand Dollars ($500,000) in the aggregate. DENTIST shall provide ABC and/or any group covered under Benefit Agreement to ABC with a Certificate of Insurance providing at least thirty (30) days' cancellation notice to ABC as evidence of compliance with this Part. The Certificate of Insurance shall be provided to ABC within forty-five (45) days after the yearly anniversary date of the professional liability insurance policy.

12.2 DENTIST hereby agrees to hold harmless, defend and indemnify ABC, its contracting groups, their Board of Directors, officers, or administrators, from and against all claims, lawsuits, demands, or actions that may arise out of any alleged malpractice or negligent act or omission to act, caused or alleged to have been caused by DENTIST or any of DENTIST'S agents, employees, consultants, associates, owners, or partners in the performance or omission of any professional duty assumed by the DENTIST pursuant to this Contract. This obligation to save and hold harmless and indemnify ABC shall be inclusive of all dental services performed whether scheduled under one of the ABC plans, under any amendment thereto, under any new plan in which DENTIST participates or whether the services are to be paid by the Member.

12.3 LITIGATION: Should ABC or any of its contracting organizations be forced to defend itself in any lawsuit, claim, demand, or action for any malpractice, negligence, or liability on the part of DENTIST, except when such actions arise as a result of a decision promulgated by ABC's Peer Review Committee, Public Policy Committee or denial of authorization or restriction of treatment by the Dental Director, DENTIST hereby agrees to provide legal counsel and shall be responsible for the cost of the defense. Should DENTIST fail to procure adequate counsel to the satisfaction of ABC, ABC may employ its own attorney(s) and DENTIST agrees to pay the cost.

PART 13. ASSIGNMENT OF CONTRACT

13.1 This Contract, being intended to secure the personal services of the DENTIST and Dentists in association with the

> **CAUTION — WATCH YOUR STEP**

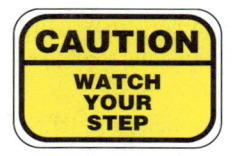

DENTIST, shall not be assigned or transferred or its duties delegated without the written consent of ABC consistent with Part 17 (Special Notice).

> *Actually, ABC's plan will allow you to use associates. Others may not! Always scrutinize the "assignment" section(s)!*

13.2 Terminating this Contract effective on the date of sale; or

13.2-1 Assigning this Contract to the purchaser of the DENTIST'S practice.

13.3 Notwithstanding ABC's options, DENTIST shall remain liable for any and all damages, injuries, or claims sustained by ABC if DENTIST fails to notify ABC as required by this Part 13.

PART 14. CLAIMS AGAINST MEMBERS

DENTIST agrees that whether or not there is any unresolved dispute for payment claimed by DENTIST, under no circumstances will DENTIST, his/her agent, employees, consultants, specialists, or representatives, whether or not employed directly or indirectly by DENTIST, make any charges or claims against a Member for any services rendered or for which it is intended by this Contract that DENTIST will be compensated in the manner stated herein by ABC, except for any charge which is, according to the provision of this Contract, to be made directly to and be paid directly by the Member.

PART 15. DENTAL DIRECTOR

15.1 A Dental Director shall be appointed by ABC to assist with the establishment of a Standard of Care, monitor the quality of care, interpret the scope of the Covered Dental Services, and serve as liaison with all Dentists.

15.2 The Dental Director shall designate and approve the forms, including quality control forms, specialist referral forms, treatment encounter forms, quarterly reports, and methods of collection of statistical professional data. DENTIST hereby agrees to use such forms and follow all such policies as promulgated by ABC concerning the use and completion of such forms.

15.3 The Dental Director shall promulgate policies and procedures as may be necessary and shall communicate the policies and procedures to DENTIST by special notice. DENTIST acknowledges that he/she has received and read the policies and procedures and agrees to follow them. DENTIST has thirty (30) days to appeal these changes with special notice as in 11.7.

15.4 The Dental Director will appoint a Dental Peer Review Committee of licensed Dentists who shall advise and assist the Dental Director in the supervision of Standards of Care, matters which relate to the DENTIST/patient relationship, interpretation of the Covered Dental Services and Benefit Agreement, or other matters involving problems within the scope of dental ethics. Prior to making a decision affecting a particular Dentist or practice, such Dentist or practice shall be granted a hearing before the Peer Review Committee and be given an opportunity to present facts in the case. The decision of the Dental Director and/or the Peer Review Committee on such matters shall be final and binding on the parties hereto, subject to a Member's final appeal to ABC's Public Policy Committee.

PART 16. TERMINATION OF CONTRACT

16.1 This Contract may be terminated by ABC with fifteen (15) days' Special Notice for cause for violation of any of the following provisions of this Contract by DENTIST:

Appendix II

        16.1-1   Failure to schedule appointments as provided herein

        16.1-2   Failure to cooperate with the Dental Director and/or the Peer Review Committee

        16.1-3   Failure to maintain the Standard of Care required herein

        16.1-4   Failure to offer Covered Dental Services to plan Members

        16.1-5   Failure to follow Specialty Referral Guidelines

16.2   At any time during the term of this Contract, ABC or DENTIST may give sixty (60) days' written Special Notice to the other party to terminate this Contract with or without cause. This contract will be terminated with or **without cause** sixty (60) days following the first day of the following month following the receipt of the Special Notice by the other party to this Contract.

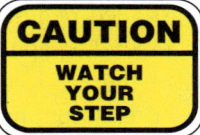

> **CAUTION — WATCH YOUR STEP**

> This will be a difficult point to negotiate away, but try — termination without cause is rarely in the provider's best interest.

16.3   This Contract may be terminated immediately by either party, if any of the following events occur:

        16.3-1   Any of the capitation payments provided by Part 5 of this Contract are not paid within fifteen (15) days after Special Notice by the DENTIST.

        16.3-2   ABC or DENTIST is no longer able to legally perform the obligations set forth in this Contract.

        16.3-3   The death of the DENTIST

        16.3-4   DENTIST becomes disabled so as to be unable to perform the obligations set forth in this Contract.

16.3-5   DENTIST is no longer licensed to practice within the state.

16.4   In the event of the termination of this Contract, DENTIST shall complete work started prior to the termination date as follows:

16.4-1   If an impression has been taken, DENTIST will complete and place the crown, bridge, partial, or denture within sixty (60) days.

16.4-2   Single tooth multivisit procedures within thirty (30) days.

16.5   In the event of termination of this Contract, DENTIST agrees to forward to the Member's new assigned dentist, at the request of the Member, the records and radiographs of the Member, within thirty (30) days of the request. DENTIST shall be reimbursed for the actual costs of any record or radiograph duplication.

16.6   In the event this Contract is terminated for any reason specified herein, DENTIST shall not render professional service to any ABC Member after the effective date of the termination other than specified in Part 16.4 of this Contract. In the event DENTIST does render professional care, DENTIST shall be fully responsible for all charges for professional services excepting therefrom any applicable co-payment for which Member will be responsible. DENTIST shall in all other respects treat the Member as if the DENTIST was still an ABC provider notwithstanding the Contract termination.

> **CAUTION — WATCH YOUR STEP**
>
> This provision puts you on the hook for any procedures that do not involve patient co-payments.

16.7   In the event of termination of the Contract for any reason, DENTIST shall be paid the last monthly capitation check due as specified in Part 4 hereof by the forty-fifth (45) day

Appendix II

following the effective date of termination of this Contract as specified therein.

PART 17. SPECIAL NOTICE

17.1 Whenever it shall become necessary for either party to serve notice on the other party with respect to this Contract, notice shall be in writing and shall be served by Certified Mail, Return Receipt Requested, to the administrative office of ABC Dental Plan, Inc., or if such notice is initiated by ABC, to the practice address on file of the DENTIST.

PART 18. ARBITRATION

18.1 Should any dispute, grievance, or controversy of any kind or nature arise between the parties to this Contract involving this Contract or any of its terms and conditions, its breach or nonperformance, the dispute, grievance, or controversy shall be submitted to binding arbitration in accordance with the rules and regulations of the American Arbitration Association. Judgment upon the award rendered by the Arbitrator may be duly entered in any court in the state having jurisdiction thereof. The Arbitrator shall have no power to change or amend this Contract.

18.2 The costs of arbitration shall be shared equally by the parties, but each party shall be responsible for the costs of its own case preparation and presentation. However, if either party considers the arbitration to be frivolous or so substantially without merit as to be considered harassment, the defending party may request and the Arbitrator may award to the party an amount not to exceed the party's cost of defending such frivolous charges.

Part 19. Miscellaneous

19.1 ABC shall have the right to use the name of the DENTIST for purposes of informing Members and prospective Members of the identity of DENTIST and his/her practice location. ABC and DENTIST each reserve the right to control the use of their respective names, symbols, trademarks, or service marks presently existing, or later established. In addition, neither ABC nor DENTIST shall use the other party's name in advertising or promotional materials without written consent.

19.2 This Contract represents the entire agreement between the parties hereto and supersedes any and all prior written or oral agreements, contracts, representations, or understandings.

ABC DENTAL PLAN, INC.   **DENTIST**
By _____   By _____
Title _____   Address _____
                                              City/State/ZIP _____
                                              Dental License # _____
                                              Tax ID # _____

GLOSSARY

Accessibility. Degree to which the delivery system inhibits or facilitates the ability of an individual to gain entry and to receive services (includes geographic, transportation, social, time, and financial considerations).

Administrative Costs. Those costs that are incurred for maintaining health services including paperwork, health screens to determine eligibility, claim processing, enrollment, billing, marketing, and other overhead expenses for any given health plan.

Administrative Services Only (ASO) or Administrative Services Contract (ASC). Coverage is essentially a noninsured arrangement offered by commercial carriers in which the group purchases administrative services (including claims adjudication, member services, and management information reporting) from the carrier but bears the full risk for the cost of health claims. Under ASO, the group makes funds available as needed for the administrator to pay claims.

Adverse Selection. The tendency for persons with poorer than average dental health to apply for and utilize dental plan services and benefits to a greater extent than do persons with average or better dental health/hygiene practices. Increases potential for higher-than-expected overall utilization and for costs above budgeted projection.

Affiliate. An organization or person that directly, or indirectly through one or more intermediaries, controls, is controlled by, or is under control with the contractor and that provides services from the contractor.

Aid to Families with Dependent Children (AFDC). The public assistance program that provides a cash grant and special support to children deprived of parental support or care and their eligible relatives.

Ambulatory Care. All types of health services that are provided on an outpatient basis are ambulatory care, in that the member has come to a location such as a clinic, health center, or dentist's office to receive services and has departed the same day.

Appropriate. Determination that the service being provided is suited for the condition that is present; suitable for a particular person, group, community, condition, occasion, and/or place.

Appropriateness of Care. A dental service must have a reasonable potential to enhance the health of the member.

At-Risk. Refers to any service for which the provider agrees to accept responsibility to provide or arrange for the provision of dental services in exchange for the capitation payment.

Beneficiary. Any person eligible to receive services in the program.

Benefit Booklet (also Evidence of Coverage). A booklet for the employee that contains a general explanation of benefits and related provisions of the dental plan.

Benefit Package. A listing of specific benefits provided by an employee benefit plan.

Glossary

Benefit Period. Period for application of deductibles, after which time deductible must again be satisfied.

Benefits. The amounts payable by a health plan for the cost of various covered dental services. In dental managed care, a detailed explanation of any necessary patient payment amounts, limitations, and exclusions.

Capitated Service. Any covered service for which the contractor receives capitation payment.

Capitation. A contractual arrangement through which a health-care provider agrees to provide specified health-care services to members for a fixed amount per month.

Capitation Rate. The amount paid per member, per month for services to be provided at-risk.

Case Management. The primary care dentist coordinates medically necessary quality dental care and assures continuity of care for members. This responsibility includes determination of health risk, identification of disease, development of a treatment plan, referral, consultation, follow-up care, prior approval of referred services, and coordinating and monitoring all plan-covered dental benefits. The PDC also assures that preventive services are provided in accordance with established standards of practice and periodicity schedules.

Catchment Area. The geographic area from which a particular program or facility draws the bulk of its users.

Closed Panel. A closed panel practice is established if patients eligible for dental services in a public or private program can receive these services only at specified facilities through a limited number of providers. If the services are provided in a group practice facility and are prepaid by some agency, the practice may be termed "prepaid group practice."

Coinsurance. An arrangement under which the insured pays for a stated portion of the cost of care. Ordinarily, the shares are expressed as a percentage (e.g., 80% of costs are paid by the insurer and 20% by the insured).

Concurrent Review. The process by which dental treatment involving a specific procedure or group of procedures is tracked for quality assurance reasons while the patients are in active treatment phase.

Consolidated Omnibus Budget Reconciliation Act of 1985 (COBRA). A federal law that requires employers with 20 or more employees to offer continued health insurance coverage to certain employees and their beneficiaries who have had their group health insurance terminated.

Continuity of Care. The concept that the plan of care for a particular member should progress without unreasonable interruption.

Contract. The written agreement between the dentist and the contractor (also called a provider agreement).

Contractor. A licensed entity under contract to provide medically necessary dental services under a prepaid fixed sum to specified beneficiaries within access and quality of care guidelines.

Coordination of Benefits (COB). Term used to designate the antiduplication provision that limits benefits for multiple group health insurance in a particular case to 100% of the expenses covered and to designate the order in which the multiple carriers are to pay benefits.

Co-payment. Payments made by the patient at the time dental care services are used. Co-payments are generally a set amount depending upon the specific service received (e.g., $10 for an office visit).

Cost Containment. A wide variety of strategies or methods whose primary goal is to control the rising cost of health care, thus making health care more affordable to Americans. These strategies and methods may include but are not limited to government regulation, managed-care programs, payment policies, global budgets, rate setting, consumer education, and utilization management.

Cost Sharing. The part of dental care expenses that a patient must pay, including deductibles, co-payments, coinsurance, and charges over the amount reimbursed by the dental benefits plan.

Cost Shifting. The practice of increasing revenues from one type of

Glossary

payer (e.g., privately insured patients) in order to cover the costs of uncompensated care or other shortfalls in reimbursement from other payers and dental plans.

Credentialing. The plan's determination as to the qualifications and ascribed privileges of a specific provider to render specific dental services.

Deductible. The amount an insured person must pay each year before the dental plan will make any payments for covered benefits.

Dental Director. The managed-care plan's director who is required to be a licensed D.D.S. or D.M.D. within the state in which the plan operates.

Dental Increasing Benefit Program. A dental program that pays an increasing share of the treatment cost, provided that the covered individual utilizes the benefits of the program during each incentive period (usually a year) and receives the treatment prescribed. For example, a 70%/30% co-payment program in the first year of coverage may become an 80%/20% program in the second year if the subscriber visits the dentist each year as stipulated in the program. There may be a corresponding percentage reduction in the co-payment level if the covered individual fails to visit the dentist in a given year (but never below the initial co-payment level).

Dental Insurance. Private insurance available through an individual or group plan that covers dental services.

Dental Maintenance Organization (DMO). Provides comprehensive dental services to a particular group for a fixed fee.

Disenrollment. Termination of an employee's health-care coverage, whether voluntary or involuntary.

Dual Option. Refers to federal legislation that requires employers to give their employees the option to enroll in a local HMO rather than in a traditional program.

Early and Periodic Screening, Diagnosis, and Treatment (EPSDT). A Medicaid program for participants under age 21 that pays for screening and diagnostic services to detect physical or mental problems and to provide health care (including dental services) needed to correct or ameliorate any defects or chronic conditions discovered.

Electronic Claims Submission (ECS). The application of electronic data interchange in replacing paper claims and documentation required administratively by dental plans.

Electronic Data Interchange (EDI). The communication of information between computer applications in a standard format.

Emergency Services. Those health services required for alleviation of severe pain or immediate diagnosis and treatment of unforeseen dental conditions, which if not immediately diagnosed and treated, could lead to disability or death (Welfare and Institutions Code, Section 14087).

Encounter. A dentally related service (or visit) rendered by a provider to a person who is enrolled in the plan during the date of service. It includes (but is not limited to) all services for which the plan contractor incurred any financial liability.

Enrollee. Beneficiary enrolled in contractor's plan.

Exclusionary Arrangements. Contracts that limit some or all of the principals from entering into similar agreements with competitors.

Exclusive Provider Organization (EPO). A dental benefits plan that provides benefits only if obtained through a closed panel of providers. Usually only an element of employer self-funded plans.

Federal Financial Participation. Federal expenditures provided to match state expenditures made under approved state plans.

Federally Qualified HMO. An HMO that has been determined by the federal Health Care Financing Administration to be qualified under Section 1310 (d) of the Public Health Service Act. Dental-only plans cannot be federally qualified.

Fee-for-Service. A method of reimbursement based on payment for specific services rendered to a beneficiary.

Glossary

Focused Review. A review that concentrates on a perceived problem area that may be a specific diagnosis, procedure, provider, patient, or other limited scope topic; done in lieu of a more comprehensive review or preliminary to it.

Gatekeeper. A system whereby the primary care dentist is responsible for managing all specialty referrals.

Global Budget. A cost-containment concept designed to control expenditures whereby fixed budgets are established for all providers in a given system. The United States does not currently have a global budget. In general, a global budget is tied to a universal health insurance plan that provides some form of health insurance coverage to all citizens. In countries with universal coverage that also have global budgets, providers negotiate with an administrative body to determine how to live within the limits set by the budget.

Governing Body. The governing body of the organization is the board of directors or, where the board's participation with quality improvement issues is not direct, a designated committee of the senior management of the managed-care organization.

Grievance. A complaint or disenrollment request filed by a member or provider. Grievances may be oral (informal) or written (formal).

Guidelines. A set of principles that guide dental practice by: (1) providing linkages among diagnosis, treatments, and outcomes; and (2) describing the alternatives available for each patient. Guidelines convert science-based knowledge into clinical action in a form accessible to providers, thus enabling professional judgment to inform the dental provider of preferred treatment, clarify health-care choices and their consequences for the patient, and link quality assurance and cost-effectiveness to health-care management.

Health Care Financing Administration (HCFA). An agency of the U.S. Department of Health and Human Services responsible for administering the Medicare program and overseeing the administration of state Medicaid programs.

Health Maintenance Organization (HMO). Any organization that, through a coordinated system of health care, provides or assures the delivery of an agreed upon set of comprehensive health maintenance and treatment services for an enrolled group of persons under a prepaid fixed sum. Services usually include primary care, emergency care, acute hospital care, ancillary services, extended care, and rehabilitation.

Indemnity Program. Provides specific cash payment reimbursement for specified covered services. Payments may be made either to enrollees or on assignment, directly to dental providers.

Independent Practice Association (IPA). A legal entity organized by dentists in order to collectively enter into contracts to provide dental services. The dentists must join the IPA and charge agreed-upon rates to enrolled patients, billing the association on a fee-for-service basis. The IPA may charge consumers on a capitation basis.

Indicators. These are objective, measurable, based on current knowledge and clinical experience, and used to monitor and evaluate each important aspect of care and service identified.

LEPEAT. An acronym which stands for "least expensive, professionally ethical, alternative treatment."

Managed Care. A comprehensive approach to the provision of prevention and primary dental care that combines clinical services and administrative procedures within an integrated, coordinated system to provide timely access to primary care and other medically necessary, quality dental services, cost effectively.

Managed Competition. A health-care delivery system in which providers and payers join together to form partnerships (not unlike managed-care partnerships) that offer health care and insurance as a single product, compete for customers, and are publicly accountable for outcomes and cost.

Management Information System (MIS). All data information collection processes and how the data elements are used in the plan during the plan administration processes. This includes all processes, whether manual or automated, for all plan administrative systems.

Glossary

Medicaid (Title XIX). The program authorized by Title XIX of the Social Security Act of 1965 to provide dental benefits for certain low-income persons.

Medicare (Title XVIII). The program authorized by Title XVIII of the Social Security Act of 1965 to provide payment for health services to the population age 65 and older.

Member. A beneficiary enrolled in a contractor's plan.

Mixed Model. A managed-care plan using more than one type of delivery system, such as a DMO that has both a plan-owned clinic and a separate network of providers operating out of their own offices.

Occupational Safety and Health Act (OSHA). A federal statute establishing national standards for health and safety conditions in the workplace. Enforced by the Labor Department, the act also provides for the reporting and compiling of statistics pertaining to occupational illnesses and injuries. OSHA also refers to the federal Occupational Safety and Health Administration.

Open Panel. A managed-care plan that contracts with dentists who operate out of their own offices.

Other Health Coverage. A term used to identify private individual or group dental insurance.

Outcomes. The results of the dental care process, involving either the member or provider of care, and measured at any specified point in time. Outcomes can be dental, economic, or societal in nature.

Outcomes Research. The systematic study of the relationships between health care and patient outcomes. It evaluates the outcomes, effectiveness, and appropriateness of alternative strategies for the prevention, diagnosis, treatment, and management of dental health conditions (not individual treatments).

Out-of-Area Benefits (DMO). Those benefits that the plan supplies to its enrollees when outside the geographical limits of the DMO. These benefits usually are limited to emergency dental services only.

Outpatient Care. Treatment provided to a member who is not admitted to a hospital or a health-care facility.

Overtreatment. Providing more services than are consistent with or justified by diagnosis and treatment plan; being neither necessary nor appropriate; often used with (or synonymous to) overutilization.

Peer Review. A mechanism in quality assurance and utilization review through which care delivered by dentists is reviewed by a panel of dentists.

Percentile. A range of a distribution of provided charges determined by a third-party payer for specific dental services. For example, if the third party uses an 80th percentile, maximum payment may be made for any charge at or below that level.

Personal Injury (PI). This is a program designed to recover the cost of medical services from an action involving the tort liability of a third party.

P Factor (P7). The grade of service for a telephone system. The digit following the "P" (e.g., 7) indicates the number of calls per 100 that are or can be blocked from the system. In this sample, P7 means 7 calls in 100 may be blocked, so the system is designed to meet this criterion. Typically, the grade of service is designed to meet the peak busy hour, the busiest hour of the busiest day of the year. Dental managed-care plans use this factor to judge when telephone staffing levels should be altered.

PHP. Prepaid health plans.

Point of Service Plan. Members do not have to choose how to receive services until services are needed. In some plans, members decide whether to use a PPO or an outside provider. Although the services of the outside provider are covered, benefits are greater if members select a preferred provider.

Practice Parameters. Strategies for patient management designed to assist dentists in clinical decision making. Parameters include standards, guidelines, practice options, practice advisories, and other patient-management strategies. Practice parameters may identify a range of appropriate strategies for the management of specific clinical conditions or may specify a range of appropriate uses of specific diagnostic or therapeutic interventions.

Preferred Provider Organization (PPO). A variation of traditional fee-for-service care arrangements representing dentists that contract with dental plans to provide members with services at a discounted rate. Employees have a choice among the dentists in a PPO arrangement and are not prevented from seeing a dentist outside of the PPO, but the benefit level will be lowered.

Preventive Care. Treatment designed to prevent dental disease or its consequences. Preventive care services include, but are not necessarily limited to, examination, diagnosis, and treatment planning; fluoridation of community water supplies; oral prophylaxis and application of topical fluorides and sealants; dietary fluoride supplements; restoration of carious teeth; maintenance of space resulting from the early loss of primary teeth; and patient education. Preventive services are provided in accordance with established periodicity schedules.

Primary Care. The basic level of dental care usually rendered by general practitioners. This type of care emphasizes caring for the member's general dental needs as opposed to a more episodic or fragmented approach to dental care.

Primary Care Dentist. A dentist responsible for supervising, coordinating, and providing initial and primary care to patients; initiating referrals for specialty care; and maintaining the continuity of patient care.

Prior Authorization. Also known as "preauthorization" or "approval," this is authorization granted by a dental managed-care plan in advance of the rendering of a service after appropriate dental review.

Process Measures of Quality. Measures of the activity of dentists in caring for patients. To evaluate providers' performance, it is valid to use only process measures that have been shown to improve or harm patients' oral health and satisfaction.

Providers. This describes a range of health-care professionals or organizations that deliver health-care services.

Quality Assessment. A limited measure of the quality of care within a particular setting.

Quality Assurance. The measurement of the quality of care and the implementation of any necessary changes to either maintain or improve the quality of care rendered.

Quality of Care. The degree to which dental services are delivered in accordance with established professional standards of structure, process, and outcome.

Reinsurance. Coverage secured by the contractor that limits the amount of liability or risk assumed under this contract.

Relative Value Unit (RVU). The linking of procedures to unit values defined by the time, skill, and costs incurred during treatment.

Retroactive Review. Traditional form of utilization review. Dental provider profiles are analyzed from submitted claims, and "outliers" can be subject to individual review.

Scope of Care. An inventory of clinical activities. A delineated scope of care provides a basis for identifying those aspects of care that will be the focus of monitoring and evaluating activities of the internal quality assurance plan.

Scope of Services. Those specific dental services for which a provider has been credentialed (by the plan) to provide to members.

Self-Insured Plan. A health-care program in which employers fund benefit plans from their own resources without purchasing them from a carrier. Self-funded plans may be self-administered, or the employer may contract with an outside administrator for administrative services only.

Service Area. The geographic area comprised of those areas designated by the U.S. Postal Service zip codes that insure adequate access to health care services by the plan members who reside therein.

Service Location. Any location at which a member obtains any health-care service provided by the contractor under the terms of the contract.

Service Site. The location designated by the contractor at which members receive primary care dentist services.

Specialty Boards. Dental administrative bodies that regulate specialty fields of dentistry by maintaining quality of care and board recognition of dentists who successfully pass certification examinations.

Specialty Care. Specialized dental care necessary to supplement primary care to meet members' needs. Requires the knowledge of a dentist who is a specialist.

Stop-Loss Coverage. Insurance purchased by a dental plan from an insurance company to reimburse the plan for the costs of benefits paid for an individual enrollee or an insurance account in excess of a stated amount. Also referred to as "reinsurance."

Subcontract. An agreement entered into between the contractor and the subcontractor for any services necessary to meet the requirements of the contract.

Subcontractor. A dentist or institution that contracts with the contractor to provide covered, medically necessary dental services.

Third-Party Administrator (TPA). An independent person or corporate entity who administers group benefits, claims, and administration for a self-insured company/group. The TPA does not insure (or accept) any risk.

Threshold. A benchmarking process for each indicator.

Traditional Indemnity Plans. In these fee-for-service group health insurance plans, the patient chooses any licensed dentist or participating provider. The employer pays premiums to the dental plan to cover the costs of providing benefits and administering claims. The employee may pay a portion of the monthly premium, annual deductible, and/or co-payment per dental visit. These plans are usually experience-rated, and dentists are paid on a cost-related, retroactive reimbursement system. The dental plan uses the premiums to pay claims, retention fees, state taxes, administrative expenses, commissions, risk charges, and claims processing. The employer (purchaser) has no liability for any deficit.

Undertreatment. Failure to recommend at the proper time one or more of those services that, consistent with diagnosis and treatment planning, are necessary and appropriate.

Universal Health Care. The availability of adequate health insurance with equal access to appropriate health-care services in a system that covers all persons living in a country or other geographic area.

Urgent Care. Services required to prevent serious deterioration of health following the onset of an unforeseen condition or injury.

Utilization. The rate patterns of service usage or types of service occurring within a specified time.

Utilization Review. The process of evaluating the necessity, appropriateness, and efficiency of the use of dental services, procedures, and facilities.

Vertical Integration. A merger of entities in a purchaser-supplier relationship.

Waivers. In order to pursue certain health-care reform measures, states need to secure authorizations to deviate from specified federal laws and regulations. These authorizations are known as "waivers."

REFERENCES

1. National Association of Prepaid Dental Plans, personal correspondence, 8 June 1994.

2. The White House Domestic Policy Council, *The President's Health Security Plan* (New York: Times Books, 1993).

3. California Dental Association, "Los Angeles United School District Study" (May 1993).

4. California Department of Health Services, "Expanding Medi-Cal Managed Care" (March 1993).

5. American Dental Association, *Report of the Practice Parameters Management Committee* (1991).

6. F.S. Foti, "Parameters of Care," *AGD Impact* 22, no. 3 (1994).

7. American Dental Association, op. cit.

8. Albert Guay, D.D.S., "Managed Dental Care—Coming Soon to Your

Neighborhood," *Connecticut State Dental Association Journal* (Spring 1991): 21.

9. "Treatment Guidelines under Development to Address Cost, Quality of Minnesota's Dental Care," *PR Newswire,* 23 November 1993.

10. Don Shuwarger, M.D., electronic personal communication, ©16 June 1994, Don Shuwarger.

11. Max Schoen, D.D.S., "Capitation in Dentistry: Original Concepts and Current Reality," *Journal of Public Health Policy* 12 (Summer 1991).

12. "ADA House of Delegates Resolution #42H-1993," *ADA News* 7 February 1994.

13. "Dental Health Coalition Pitched," *CDA Update* 15 February 1994.

14. Ibid.

15. Hawaii Department of Human Services, "Request for Proposal for QUEST Dental Plan" (1993): 7–9.

16. California Department of Health Services, "Expanding Medi-Cal Managed Care" (March 1993): i.

17. "Prepaid Dental Plans at Odds with ADA over Managed Care Definition," *Managed Care Report* (4 February 1991): 4.

18. "How Procedures Become Benefits," *Delta Dental Plan of New Jersey Newsletter* 20, no. 1 (March 1989).

19. O. Mitra, *Fundamentals of Quality Control and Improvement* (New York: Macmillan Publishing, 1993).

20. Maxwell Davis, D.D.S. and Benjamin Schechter, D.D.S., "The Dentist and Prepaid Capitated Systems," *Dental Clinics of North America* 31, no. 2. (April 1987).

21. Title 13, Section 4004, *Medicare Statutes of Social Security Act: Health Care Financing Administration* (March 1994).

22. Ibid., Section 4004.2.

References

23. Ibid., Section 4004.3.

24. Ibid., Section 4004.4.

25. Evelyn Ireland, executive director of the National Association of Prepaid Dental Plans (NAPDP), personal correspondence, 9 June 1994.

26. American Dental Association, *Glossary of Dental Benefit Terms* (Chicago: American Dental Association, 1993).

27. American Dental Association, Bureau of Economic and Behavioral Research, personal correspondence, March 1994.

28. "Dental HMOs Expand Enrollment and Office Space," *The Phoenix Business Journal* 13, no. 31 (4 June 1993).

29. W.M. Pollock, "Managed Care: Succeeding under Capitation," *Medical Group Management Journal* 40, no. 4 (July/August 1993): 6-7.

30. Richard B. Ryan, "Managed Care—The Real Issues and Real Problems," *Dental Economics* (January 1994).

31. American Dental Association, *Designing Your Dental Benefits Plan: A Complete Guide for Employers* (1991).

32. Daniel S. Greenberg, "Uncelebrated Triumph of Dental Health (Report on Dental Health in the U.S. Receives Little Fanfare)," *The Lancet* 340, no. 885 (8 August 1992):359 (2) (Viewpoint article).

INDEX

A

Academy of General Dentistry, 8
Acceptability/public policy, 144–145
Access to dental care, 40–41, 94–95, 142–144
Accountability, 6–7
Accreditation Association for Ambulatory Health Care, 50
Acknowledgment/disposition (grievance process), 151
Active role in managed care, 92
Administrative costs, 58
Adverse selection risk, 15, 23
Affordable Health Care Now Act of 1993, 28
Agreements/contracts, 113–123
Allied health personnel, 148
Allowances/benefits schedule, 17
American Academy of Oral & Maxillofacial Surgery, 57
American Academy of Pediatric Dentistry, 57
American Accreditation Program, Inc., 50
American Association of Endodontics, 57
American Board of Quality Assurance and Utilization Review Physicians, 47, 50
American Dental Association, 7–8, 30–32, 40, 52–53, 71, 84, 114, 121, 139, 142: health care position, 31–32
American Health Security Act of 1993, 28

Index

ANSI 837 standard, 65
ANSI/ASQC Standard A# (1987), 50
Any willing provider concept, 85–86
Application process (managed care program), 72, 76–83
Application process (provider networks), 72, 76–83
Appointment, 144
Arbitration, 120, 191–192
Arizona v. Maricopa County Medical Society, 84
Assignment of patients, 106–107
Assignment/delegation of provider, 121
At-risk contract, 22–24
Auditing, 83, 111–112, 146–147

B

Beneficiary's statement, 60
Benefit changes without consent, 103
Benefit plan standards, 141–142
Beta risk, 23
Billing for non-covered services, 102–103
Billing forms, 103–104
Board of Dental Examiners, 98
Broken appointment (follow-up), 145

C

California Dental Association, 2, 8, 32, 47, 53, 109, 142
California Department of Corporations, 41, 47, 141
California Department of Health Services, 38–39
Capacity (patient), 108–109
Capitation program, 16, 20–24, 36–37, 101, 115–116: at-risk contract, 22–24
Care audit, 146–147
Care rendition (provider agreement), 176–178
Care review system (quality of), 146–148
Caries prevention, 157
Case management, 56–57
CDC guidelines, 56
Chicago (IL) public schools, 9–10
Claims against members, 187
Claims volume, 59
Clark v. Coye, 41
Cleanliness, 149
Clinton administration, x, 27
Clinton Health Security Plan (1993)/Health Care Act, 28–30
Communication, 143
Computerization of records/resources, 99
Consumer Choice Health Security Act of 1993, 28
Contacts, 91
Continuity (of care), 145
Continuous quality improvement, xi, 45
Contract assignment, 186–187
Contract modifications, 118
Contract termination, 188–191

Contract (term of), 182
Coordinated case management, xi
Co-payments, 116
Corrective action plan, 56, 82
Cost containment, 17–18, 38, 47–48
Cost-effective dental practice, 97–99
Cost-effectiveness (treatment), 96–97
Cost-shifting paradigm, 27
Council on Dental Care Programs (ADA), 9
Coverage (dental services), 116
Credentialing, xi
Crown/fixed partial prosthodontics, 165–167

D

Dade County (FL) public schools, 10
Definitions (provider agreement), 174–176
Delta Dental Plan, xi–xii, 9, 30, 50, 66
Demand risk, 23
Dental assistant, 98
Dental benefits, 15, 30, 33–34: in health-care reform, 33–34
Dental care standard, 182–183
Dental director, 187–188
Dental Health Coalition, 30, 32–33
Dental hygienist, 98
Dental labs policy, 107–108

Dental maintenance organizations, 24–25, 68. *See also* Managed care in dentistry.
Dental Managed Care Unit (CDHS), xi
Dental plans, 14–25: payment based on UCR fees, 16–17; allowances/benefits schedule, 17; cost containment, 17–18; fee-for-service plans, 17–18; direct reimbursement, 18; preferred provider organizations, 19–20; exclusive provider organizations, 20; capitation-based programs, 20–22; capitation and at-risk contract, 22–24; dental maintenance organizations, 24–25
Dental program mixture, 135
Dental provider agreement (sample), 173–192
Dental provider's statement, 60–61
Dental records, 146
Dental services in core benefits, 34–35
Dental specialist, 87–92, 143: concerns of, 87–92; marketing, 90; referrals, 90; contacts, 91; multispecialty practice, 91; subspecializing, 91–92; active role in managed care, 92
Denti-Cal, xii, 41
Dentist extenders, 98
Dentist name use, 192
Dentist-patient relationship, 184–185
Denture prosthodontics (complete), 168–170
Diagnosis, 155

Index

Direct reimbursement, 18
Direct service contracts, 72–76
Discrimination (grievance process), 151
Disease prevention/diagnosis/treatment, 28–29, 34
Dispute resolution, 122
Diversification, 135
DMO. *See* Dental maintenance organizations.
Documentation (grievance process), 151
Dropouts/terminations from program, 133–137: provider agreement language, 134; performance evaluation criteria, 135; dental program mixture, 135; network with employers, 135; independent practice association, 136; response to termination, 136–137

E

Early and Periodic Screening, Diagnosis, and Treatment, 30
Electronic claims submission, 65
Electronic data interchange, 55, 65–66
Electronic funds transfer, 66
Eligibility (provider agreement), 178–179
Emergency care/services, 28, 34, 41–42
Employee satisfaction, 2–3
Encounter data reporting, 21, 55, 58–66: beneficiary's statement, 60; dental provider's statement, 60–61; definition, 61–63; utilization review systems, 62, 64–65; electronic data interchange, 65–66
Endodontics, 88, 158–161
Enrollee information, 143
Equipment licensure, 148
Ethnic group, 42
Excluded procedures/services, 116–117
Exclusive provider organizations, 20
External auditing, 111–112

F

Facility/personnel/equipment licensure, 148–149
Fee schedule, 84
Fee-for-service, 2–3, 5, 17–18, 54, 120, 127, 132
Financial aspects monitoring, 99
First Annual Dental Managed Care Congress (1994), 105
Format/records/files (grievance procedure), 150
Fractional practice analysis, 114, 124–132: relative value unit, 127; procedure for, 127–132

G

Glossary of terms, 193–206
Grievance system/process, 55–56, 110–111, 119, 150–151
Group practice (provider network), 69

H

HCFA-1500, 65
Health-care costs, 3
Health Care Financing Administration, 47, 68
Health Care Quality Improvement Act of 1986, 53, 109–110
Health-care reform, 26–35: Clinton Health Security Plan/Health Care Act, 28–30; American Dental Association health-care position, 31–32; Dental Health Coalition, 32–33; dental benefits in health-care reform, 33–34; dental services in core benefits, 34–35; future strategies, 35
Health Equity and Access Reform Today Act of 1993, 28
Health Insurance Association of America, 39
Health maintenance organizations, ix–xii, 11, 67–68. *See also* Dental maintenance organizations *and* Managed care in dentistry.
History/clinical examination, 151–153
HMO. *See* Health maintenance organizations.
HMO Act of 1973, 68
Hold-harmless clauses, 118

I

Illegal contract of adhesion, 134
Independent practice association, 68, 72, 136

Indian Dental Association of California, 42
Individual practice association, 69–71, 82, 84–85
Infection control, 56
Insurance, 120
Integrated Service Networks (Minnesota), 9
International Classification of Diseases (ICD-9) codes, 52
International Longshoremen's Union, 20

J

Jackson Hole Group, 26–27
Joint Commission on Accreditation of Healthcare Organizations, 50

K

Knox-Keene dental guidelines, 141–172: regulations, 142–151; accessibility, 142–144; acceptability/public policy, 144–145; continuity of care, 145; care review, 146–148; facility/personnel/equipment licensure, 148–149; grievance system, 150–151; quality of care, 151–172; history/clinical examination, 151–153; radiographs, 153–155; diagnosis, 155; treatment planning, 156–157; preventive dentistry, 157–158; endodontics, 158–161; periodontics, 161–163; oral and maxillofacial surgery, 163–167;

removable partial prosthodontics, 167–168; complete denture prosthodontics, 168–170; pedodontics, 170; orthodontics, 171–172

Knox-Keene Health Care Service Plan Act, 141

Korean Dentists of the USA, 42

L

Legal considerations (provider networks), 85–86

LEPEAT principle, 97

Liability/liability insurance, 24, 185–186

Licensing. *See* Facility/personnel/equipment licensure.

Limitations of coverage, 29

Linguistic/cultural sensitivities, 42

Liquidated damages, 121

Loss-leader strategy, 19

M

Managed care in dentistry, ix–xii, 9–10, 36–48: access, 40–41; service area, 41; emergency services, 41–42; linguistic/cultural sensitivities, 42; provider network, 42–43; referral system, 43–45; quality assurance program, 45–47; cost containment, 47–48. *See also* Dental maintenance organizations *and* Managed care in your practice.

Managed care in your practice, 93–99: access to dental care, 94–95; quality dental care, 95–96; cost-effectiveness of treatment, 96–97; cost-effective dental practice, 97–99. *See also* Managed care in dentistry.

Managed Competition Act of 1993, 28

Management information systems, 59, 110

Marketing, 90

Maximum patient capacity, 108–109

Medicaid/Medicare, 27

Medi-Cal Dental Managed Care Program, xii

Medical emergency preparedness, 149

Mercury safety, 149

Mixed models (provider networks), 71

Monitoring system (accessibility), 142

Most-favored nation clause, 120

Multispecialty practice, 91

N

National Aerospace and Space Administration, 11

National Association of Prepaid Dental Plans, xii, 89

National Board of Medical Examiners, 51

National Committee on Quality Assurance, 47, 50

National Practitioner Data Bank, 53–54, 109–110

Netherlands, 65

Networking with employers, 135
Noncompetition clauses, 120–121
Nonexclusive contract, 183
Nonsurgical root canal treatment, 160

O

Occupational Safety and Health Administration, 142
Oral and maxillofacial surgery, 163–167
Oral disease prevention, 158
Oral health, 98–99
Orthodontics, 29–30, 171–172
OSHA. *See* Occupational Safety and Health Administration.
OSHA compliance/infection control, 56

P

Patient assignment, 106–107
Patient eligibility, 104
Patient-load capacity, 108–109
Patient/provider grievances, 55–56
Payment frequency, 102
Payment to dentist (basis of), 180
Payment (UCR fees), 16–17
Pediatrics, 89
Pedodontics, 170
Peer review, 53–54, 109–110, 146

Performance evaluation criteria, 135
Periodontal disease prevention, 157
Periodontics, x–xi, 34, 88, 161–163
Personnel licensure/certification, 148
PHP. *See* Prepaid health plans.
Point-of-service plans, 24–25
Practice profiles, 53–55, 62
Preferred provider organizations, 11, 19–20, 88
Prepaid health plans, 141
Preventive dentistry, 157–158
Preventive measure (oral and maxillofacial surgery), 163–164
Price risk, 23
Primary care dentist, 38, 43–45, 70, 88, 90, 98, 118–119
Principal limitations, 117
Privileging, xi
Professional risk, 24
Prostheses, 165–170
Provider agreement language, 134
Provider agreements/contracts, 113–123: reimbursement, 114–117; important elements, 117–123; terms/conditions, 117–118; contract modifications, 118; hold-harmless clauses, 118; referrals, 118–119; utilization review, 119; grievance system, 119; arbitration, 120; insurance, 120; most-favored nation clause, 120; noncompetition

Index

clauses, 120–121; assignment/delegation, 121; liquidated damages, 121; rules/policies, 122; state of jurisdiction, 122; risk pools/withholds/bonuses, 122; stop-loss arrangements, 122–123

Provider complaints/grievances/appeals, 110–111

Provider networks, 42–43, 67–86: staff model, 68–69; group practice, 69; individual practice associations, 69–71, 82, 84–85; mixed models, 71; direct service contracts, 72–76; application process, 72, 76–83; legal considerations, 85–86

Provider termination, 104–105, 133–137

Public policy. *See* Acceptability/public policy.

Q

Quality assurance and managed care, 49–57: quality assurance program, 53–57; peer review, 53–54; utilization review, 54–55; patient/provider grievances, 55–56; OSHA compliance/infection control, 56; case management, 56–57

Quality assurance program, 45–47, 49–57, 111–112, 142

Quality of care, 95–96, 142, 151–172: guidelines, 142

QUEST (Hawaii), 37–38

Questions for prospective plans, 100–112: reimbursement determination, 101; payment frequency, 102; billing for noncovered services, 102–103; benefit changes without consent, 103; billing forms, 103–104; patient eligibility, 104; termination, 104–105; renegotiation of agreement, 106; assignment of patients, 106–107; dental labs policy, 107–108; maximum patient capacity, 108–109; peer review system, 109–110; records inspection, 110; provider complaints/grievances/appeals, 110–111; external auditing, 111–112

R

Radiography, 54, 66, 148–149, 153–155: safety, 148–149

Records inspection, 110

Referrals/referral system, 43–45, 90, 118–119, 143, 145

Reform strategies (health care), 35

Regulation/regulatory agency, 141–144

Reimbursement, 18, 101, 114–117, 125–126

Relative value unit, 101, 127, 129–130

Removable partial prosthodontics, 167–168

Renegotiation of agreement, 106

Response to termination, 136–137

Responsibility (grievance process), 150–151
Restoration, 34, 165–170
Risk pools/withholds/bonuses, 122
Root canal treatment, 159–161
Rules/policies, 122

S

Safety plan, 148
Safety (radiology), 148–149
Service area (geography), 41
Service not covered (fee due), 179
Space maintenance procedures, 29
Special concerns. *See* Dental specialist, concerns of.
Special notice, 191
Specialist/substitute, 180–181
Specialty compensation, 89
Specialty providers, 98
Staff education/training, 97
Staff model (provider network), 68–69
Staffing pattern, 143
State of jurisdiction, 122
Sterilization/disinfection, 149
Stop-loss arrangements, 122–123
Subscriber/enrollee notification, 150
Subspecializing, 91–92
Supportive care (oral and maxillofacial surgery), 164–165
Surgical root canal treatment, 160–161

T

Tangible net equity, 102
Tax deductibility, 31–33
Temporomandibular joint therapy, 17
Term/benefit change, 182
Termination, 104–105
Terms/conditions (contracts), 117–118
Texas Department of Insurance, 12
Texas Medical Association, 12–13
Therapeutic measure (oral and maxillofacial surgery), 164
Total quality management, xi, 45
Treatment in progress clause, 117–118
Treatment planning, 156–157
Turnkey network, 84

U

UCR fees, 16–17
Upselling, 116–117
Utilization review, 54–55, 62, 64–65, 119, 148
Utilization Review Accreditation Commission, 50
Utilization risk, 23

V

Vital pulp treatment, 34, 158–159

X

X-ray equipment, 148–149